Creating Healthy and Sustainable Buildings

Mateja Dovjak · Andreja Kukec

Creating Healthy and Sustainable Buildings

An Assessment of Health Risk Factors

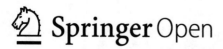
Springer Open

Mateja Dovjak
Faculty of Civil and Geodetic Engineering
University of Ljubljana
Ljubljana, Slovenia

Andreja Kukec
Faculty of Medicine, Centre of Public Health
University of Ljubljana
Ljubljana, Slovenia

ISBN 978-3-030-19414-7   ISBN 978-3-030-19412-3   (eBook)
https://doi.org/10.1007/978-3-030-19412-3

Technical editing: Tanja Rejc, National Institute of Public Health, Ljubljana, Slovenia

Illustrator: Jurij Mikuletič

This Springer imprint is published by the registered company Springer Nature Switzerland AG.
The registered company address is: Gewerbestrasse 11, 6330 Cham, Switzerland

For Sven and Borut.

Mateja Dovjak

For Lan and Aleš.

Andreja Kukec

Preface

The stock of buildings in the European Union is relatively old, with more than 40% of it built before 1960 and 90% before 1990. About 75% of the buildings are energy inefficient. According to legislation on energy efficiency, strategic action plans for the improvement of the energy performance of buildings have been accepted. However, current activities are mainly focused on increasing the thermal performance of building envelope systems, building airtightness, and energy-efficient mechanical systems. Such unilateral design of built environments results in uncomfortable and unhealthy conditions as well as other adverse health outcomes. Epidemiological studies show that approximately 30% of new and renovated buildings worldwide may be related to unhealthy indoor environments. Studies on residential buildings in Japan and in three northern European cities identified 12–30.8% of occupants as having sick building syndrome symptoms. Moreover, in the studies on public buildings in Canada, the UK, and the US, 20–50% of workers experienced sick building syndrome symptoms. Finally, statistical data show that 15.1% of Europeans live in dwellings with leaking roofs, damp walls, floors, or foundations.

Most of our exposure-related human activities are performed in indoor built environments, living as well as active working spaces. From 60 to 90% of the time spent indoors, we are exposed to numerous environmental health risk factors. Epidemiological studies define more than 23 health risk parameters related to indoor built environments that might cause adverse health effects on building users. Particularly sensitive to risk factors are vulnerable groups of users, possessing multiple, cumulative risk factors. The numbers of these are increasing as the population ages. Poor indoor environmental quality conditions, longer exposure times, the presence of vulnerable population groups, and increased user susceptibility may all increase the risk of adverse health effects. Prevention and control of health risk factors is the fundamental activity for the design of healthy and comfortable built environments.

Creating Healthy and Sustainable Buildings: An Assessment of Health Risk Factors is dedicated to all stakeholders involved in the design of built environments, particularly buildings as a whole or their separate parts throughout their life cycles. This scientific monograph systematically addresses the problem of inadequate indoor environmental quality and synthesizes new insights and own research results in the direction of its improvement. It gives a comprehensive overview of epidemiological studies, statistical data and user complaints that clearly demonstrate the consequences of incorrect activities in current design processes. Furthermore, the authors hope that the monograph will raise the awareness of society and indicate that this is the right time for a change toward healthier built environments. In this era of increased renovation rates, it is essential to have a work that can be used for effective prevention and control of health risk factors in all stages of design of built environments.

The scientific monograph consists of four chapters, presenting the morphology of the design of healthy built environments. In Chap. 1, a built environment as a four-dimensional space of the product, system, location, and user is introduced. The authors describe the problem of unhealthy built environments with the cause–effect relationship. The chapter concludes with a list of objectives of planning toward healthy sustainable buildings, and well-being. Chapter 2 is dedicated to understanding the conceptual differences between healthy buildings, beyond eco-friendly, green, or low-carbon buildings. It emphasizes the problem of current reimbursement strategies and plans that often define priority environments driven by economic and energetic criteria. Therefore, the chapter concludes with the definition of priority environments for renovation according to vulnerable population groups. In Chap. 3, readers, including students, experts, or the general public become familiar with the identification of health risk factors and their parameters and their role in the design of healthy built environments. Identified and classified health risk factors and their parameters are the basis for the identification of single- and multi-group interactions among them, described in Chap. 4. Following the evidence-based design approach, the monograph synthesizes with the tool developed for decision-making processes supported by short-term and long-term benefits of the presented holistic design.

The relevant topics related to the design of built environments are discussed from public health and engineering perspectives. In such a way, multidisciplinary cooperation between disciplines and professions as well as constructive communication are stimulated. Indeed, this is the main motivation for the monograph. This publication is valuable for all target groups involved in all levels of design of built environments:

- Academic levels: undergraduate, postgraduate, specialization, lifelong learning.
- Experts involved in all stages of design (building, its systems, indoor/outdoor environment): civil engineering, architects, environmental health engineering, mechanical engineering, medicine, public health experts, and environmentalists.
- General public: raising the awareness, knowledge.
- Institutions, organizations: public health, occupational health (guidelines).

- Legislative bodies: policymakers on the field of built environments (strategic and legal documents).
- Others: nongovernmental organizations, general people, and vulnerable population groups.

Ljubljana, Slovenia   Mateja Dovjak
                                                                             Andreja Kukec

Acknowledgements

Mateja Dovjak would like to express her sincere appreciation to Prof. Scient. Counc. Dr. Aleš Krainer, Arch., Prof. Dr. Masanori Shukuya, Kristina Likar, M.Sc., and Prof. Dr. Jože Krašovec.

Prof. Scient. Counc. Dr. Aleš Krainer, Arch. is a former Professor at the Faculty of Civil and Geodetic Engineering, University of Ljubljana (UL FGG), Faculty of Health Sciences UL, Head of Chair of Buildings and Constructional Complexes UL FGG (1989–2013). Prof. Aleš Krainer introduced me to the role of the individual user in built environments and is still raising my awareness and motivation toward the design of healthy buildings. Prof. Dr. Masanori Shukuya is a Professor at the Faculty of Environmental and Information Studies, Tokyo City University (FEIS-TCU) and is also a Professor at and Chairman of the Graduate Program for Environmental and Information Studies, Japan. He teaches me about exergy thinking in the framework of connective thinking approaches to better understand human-building relationships. Kristina Likar, M.Sc., is a former Professor at the Faculty of Health Sciences UL and Head of Sanitary Engineering Department (1981–1991, 2000–2006). She introduced me to the method of combining public health and engineering approaches with emphasized benefits for society. Jože Krašovec, Sc.B.D., Ph.D., Th.D. and Anth. Rel. D. is a member of The Slovenian and European Academy of Sciences and Arts, Professor of Biblical Sciences at the Faculty of Theology, University of Ljubljana. He helps me to acquire knowledge on the role of human as an individual and his values in the context of building design. Additionally, I would also like to extend my thanks to all users who have spoken openly about problems related to building design.

And, last but not least, I wish to thank my closest ones, Sven and Borut, who have appreciated me for my work and motivated me in writing this scientific monograph; for tiny, inconspicuous steps in the right direction today toward consequential enormous action for healthier built environments in our future.

Andreja Kukec would like to express her special thanks of gratitude to Prof. Dr. Lijana Zaletel-Kragelj, Prof. Dr. Ivan Eržen, and Prof. Dr. Otto Haninen.

Prof. Dr. Lijana Zaletel-Kragelj is a Professor at the Medical Faculty, University of Ljubljana. She has taught me about different epidemiological study designs and statistical approaches in the field of public health. Prof. Dr. Ivan Eržen is a Professor at the Medical Faculty, University of Ljubljana and Head of National Institute of Public Health, Slovenia. He has taught me about the impact of environmental health determinants on health. Prof. Dr. Otto Hänninen is a researcher at the National Institute for Health and Welfare, Finland, Department of Health Protection, Helsinki. He has introduced me to different assessment approaches in the field of industrial contaminated cities. I would also like to thank my Aleš and Lan.

Acknowledgements for proofreading to Mina Brajović, Romana Hudin, and Terry T. Jackson, for technical editing to Tanja Rejc and for illustrations to Jurij Mikuletič.

The authors acknowledge the financial support from the Slovenian Research Agency (research core funding No. P2-0158, Structural engineering and building physics and No. P5-0142, Bio-psycho-social context of kinesiology), Faculty of Civil Engineering and Medical Faculty, University of Ljubljana.

Acknowledgements to reviewers: Prof. Dr. Vincenc Butala (Faculty of Mechanical Engineering, University of Ljubljana, Slovenia), Assoc. Prof. Aleksandar Bulog, Ph.D. (Faculty of Medicine, University of Rijeka, Department of Health Ecology, Institute of Public Health of Primorsko-Goranska County, Health Ecological Department, Croatia), Assist. Prof. Rok Fink, Ph.D. (Sanitary Engineering Department, Faculty of Health Sciences, University of Ljubljana, Slovenia), Prof. Dr. Masanori Shukuya (Department of Restoration Ecology and Built Environment, Tokyo City University, Yokohama, Japan).

We would like to thank the staff at Springer Nature, in particular Shinjini Chatterjee, Christopher Wilby, Evelien Bakker, Bernadette Deelen-Mans, and Ram Prasad R. C., for their help and support. We would also like to thank Aleš Krulec, Institute of Public and Environmental Health, Ljubljana, Slovenia.

Mateja Dovjak
Andreja Kukec

Contribution of Reviewers

The manuscript is peer reviewed, following the double-blind reviewing procedure by the publisher. Additionally, it is reviewed by Prof. Dr. Vincenc Butala (Faculty of Mechanical Engineering, University of Ljubljana, Slovenia), Assoc. Prof. Dr. Aleksandar Bulog (Faculty of Medicine, University of Rijeka, Department of Health Ecology, Institute of Public Health of Primorsko-Goranska County, Health Ecological Department, Croatia), Assist. Prof. Rok Fink (Sanitary Engineering Department, Faculty of Health Sciences, University of Ljubljana, Slovenia), Prof. Dr. Masanori Shukuya (Department of Restoration Ecology and Built Environment, Tokyo City University, Yokohama, Japan).

Up to 90% of the time human being spends indoors; in some specific environments, such as hospitals, retirement home, etc., even more. During this time, occupants are exposed to numerous environmental health risk factors that might have adverse health effects. For effective control and prevention against health risk factors, the built environment has to be healthy and animatedly designed.

The scientific monograph systematically addresses the problem of deteriorated indoor environmental quality and reveals novel approach strategies against that. It represents an original scientific work that gives a comprehensive overview of the epidemiological studies, monographs, reports, legal documents, and standards. In the methodology of engineering design of healthy built environments, occupants are in the central point. It features knowledge of disciplines, engineering, and public health; readers become familiar with terminology and definitions. Especially the interesting and exhaustedly investigated chapter on interactions among health risk factors and decision-making process provides useful information and shows a good summary of current and future trends in research and development. It is a crucial step for effective assessment and prevention of problems in unhealthy built environment.

I strongly believe that the monograph is useful to all stakeholders involved in every stage of design of optimal built environments, indoors and outdoors, and highlights the main benefits of creating healthy and sustainable buildings. I hope that the book will encourage collaboration among different sectors as well as universities in preparation of novel programs or collaboration of existing ones in

Slovenia and worldwide. This should be our future mission, of each individual and of society.

Prof. Dr. Vincenc Butala
Faculty of Mechanical Engineering, University of Ljubljana, Slovenia
Editor-in-Chief of Strojniški vestnik—Journal of Mechanical Engineering;
member of international associations ASHRAE, REHVA
(REHVA Fellow), and ISIAQ. More than 40 years of experiences
in the research of the indoor environment, HVAC systems
energy conservation in buildings. More than 115 peer reviewed
scientific papers in the field of HVAC, rational energy usage
in buildings and indoor environment.

The scientific monograph: "Creating healthy and sustainable buildings: An assessment of health risk factors", Mateja Dovjak and Andreja Kukec as authors, is an original scientific work in the domain of sustainable development and all its positive and negative sides and healthy housing viewed from many important aspects. The book represents a very high-quality and comprehensive source of many theoretical and, on the other hand, practical examples of sources of many health problems that people may be exposed to in a narrow and wider environment in which they live and/or work. Many of today's widespread environmental illnesses have their source in environmental factors that can be of a chemical, biological, physical, and radiative nature. Housing conditions, architectural and construction standards, types of embedded materials in future residential or active buildings are always a very important factor in determining the occurrence of certain environmental illnesses. This book provides a large number of expert but also scientific examples of how to avoid many diseases, disabilities, or prevent health risks in people who live or work in such areas where they may be exposed to them. The book represents a highly qualified professional literature for all those professionals who are responsible for and involved in the adoption of key criteria that prescribe the conditions for quality construction of facilities that have always and, most importantly, will in the future represent key standards for sustainable development, especially in the field of health risk management. This work represents a quality literary upgrade to all levels of education (secondary schools, faculties, postgraduate studies, doctoral studies) and can be used during their education and professional development.

Associate Professor, Aleksandar Bulog, Ph.D.
Faculty of Medicine, University of Rijeka
Department of Health Ecology
Institute of Public Health of Primorsko-Goranska County
Health Ecological Department

Buildings in European Union are relatively old and strategies to cope with this problem are related mainly to the energy efficacy, not taking into account health of residents.

This scientific monograph represents comprehensive review in the field of built environment and health impacts. Most of the books deal with either building engineering or health issues related to indoor risk factors. However, this scientific monograph represents text on joint issues, as in real situations these two components are inseparable. It offers value as a textbook for students as well as for professionals in the field of building planners, operators, restorers, and for public health professions. The added value of this scientific monograph is interdisciplinary approach with the aim to inform the readers what the building factors that have an impact on human are and what the health outcomes are. The most important contribution is presentation of interactions among health risk factors and decision tool for stakeholders. The scientific monograph represents a good potential for being adopted by audience, as there are no books on the joined field of building and health science. A big advantage of this book is decision tool for the assessment of building group interactions with impact on human health.

Assist. Prof. Rok Fink, Ph.D.

Head of Sanitary Engineering Department, Faculty of Health Sciences

University of Ljubljana, and the author of scientific monograph

Hygienically relevant biofilms

People, either professionals or nonprofessionals, tend to forget the importance of the built environment. One reason for this is that everyone is being exposed to the built environment in his/her everyday life so that it looks nothing special to think carefully. The other reason is that the languages used by the people involved in designing the built environment are different and they are not necessarily conscious about the miscommunication caused by their respective different languages. Considering such present circumstance in general, this book is valuable for everyone involved in built-environmental design for making it better for the people to live in. This is a good reference book for a better communication for all involved in the design of built environment.

Masanori Shukuya, Ph.D.

Professor of Building Science, Tokyo City University

Yokohama Campus, and the author of Bio-Climatology

for Built Environment

Contents

1   **Introduction**   1
   1.1   Characteristics of Built Environments   1
   1.2   A Historical Background of the Built Environment............   5
   1.3   Morphology of Engineering Design of Built Environments   8
   1.4   Legal Framework   20
      1.4.1   Legal Framework Towards Energy Efficiency   20
      1.4.2   Legal Framework Towards a Healthy Environment   24
   1.5   Relevant Problems in the Built Environment, User
       Complaints..   26
   1.6   Most Common Problems in the Built Environment—
       Epidemiological Data   31
   1.7   Main Objectives of Planning   34
   References   35

2   **Health Outcomes Related to Built Environments**   43
   2.1   Healthy Versus Unhealthy Buildings   43
   2.2   Comfortable Versus Uncomfortable Conditions   48
      2.2.1   Satisfaction of Human Needs in the Built Environment
         and the Process of Homeostasis   48
      2.2.2   Overall Comfort   49
      2.2.3   Thermal Comfort...............................   51
   2.3   Wellbeing and Sustainable Buildings   53
      2.3.1   Sustainable, Eco-friendly, Green and Low Carbon
         Buildings   55
   2.4   Health Effects in the Built Environment....................   59
      2.4.1   Sick Building Syndrome Versus Building-Related
         Illness...   61
   2.5   Health Outcomes Related to Unhealthy Built Environments   63
      2.5.1   Building Dampness   64
      2.5.2   Uncomfortable Thermal Environment   65

2.5.3   Poor Indoor Air Quality   66
2.5.4   Excessive Noise   67
2.5.5   Lack of Daylight   68
2.6   Population Groups and Priority Environments   70
References   74

3   Identification of Health Risk Factors and Their Parameters   83
3.1   Determinants of Health, Health Risk, and Health Hazard
       Factors   83
3.2   Identification and Classification of Health Risk Factors
       in Built Environments and Their Parameters   87
3.3   Association Between Potential Health Outcomes and Physical
       Health Risk Factors in Built Environments   89
3.4   Association Between Potential Health Outcomes and Chemical
       Health Risk Factors in Built Environments   96
3.5   Association Between Potential Health Outcomes and Biological
       Health Risk Factors in Built Environments   103
3.6   Association Between Potential Health Outcomes and
       Psychosocial Health Risk Factors in Built Environments   108
3.7   Association Between Potential Health Outcomes and Other
       Factors in Built Environments   109
References   110

**4   Interactions Among Health Risk Factors and Decision-Making
Process in the Design of Built Environments**   121
4.1   Health Risk and Management Assessment Model in Built
       Environments   122
4.2   Single-Group Interactions   122
       4.2.1   Physical-Physical Interactions   123
       4.2.2   Chemical-Chemical Interactions   124
       4.2.3   Chemical-Physical Interactions   127
       4.2.4   Chemical-Biological Interactions   130
       4.2.5   Biological-Biological Interactions   131
       4.2.6   Biological-Physical Interactions   132
       4.2.7   Personal-Physical Interactions   134
       4.2.8   Personal-Chemical Interactions   136
       4.2.9   Interactions Between Other Health Risk Factors
                and Their Parameters   137
4.3   Multi-group Interactions   138
4.4   Decision-Making Tool in the Design of Built Environments   140
4.5   Short-Term and Long-Term Benefits of Holistic Design   145
References   148

Index   157

Chapter 1
Introduction

Abstract This chapter provides an introduction to the problems of unhealthy and uncomfortable conditions in built environments. In Sect. 1.1, the characteristics of built environments, which include living as well as working areas, is introduced. In Sect. 1.2, the historical background of built environments is described. The morphology of the engineering design of built environments supplemented by descriptions of specific requirements and needs for active spaces are presented (Sect. 1.3). Current legislation on building energy use, environmental protection, and public health strategies is listed in Sect. 1.4. Section 1.5 presents relevant problems in the built environment supported by studies and user's opinions. A comprehensive review of the epidemiological data on relevant problems in built environments is provided, as well as their causes and consequences from engineering and public health perspectives (Sect. 1.6). At the end of this chapter, in Sect. 1.7, we conclude the main objectives of planning towards healthy and sustainable buildings and general wellbeing.

1.1 Characteristics of Built Environments

The term "built environment" refers to all aspects of the human-made surroundings that provide the setting for human activity: the human-made space in which people live, work, and create on a day-to-day basis (Roof and Oleru 2008). It ranges in scale from indoor to outdoor active spaces, and it extends in four-dimensional space (i.e., length-x, width-y, depth-z, time-t), so the boundaries among them are often blurred (Fig. 1.1).

Early concepts of built environments date to Classical Antiquity; notable is the work of Hippodamus of Miletos, an architect and urban planner who lived between 498 and 408 BCE (Glaeser 2011). He is considered the father of urban planning, and his name is given to the grid layout of city planning, known as the Hippodamian plan, which is based on a grid of right angles and the allocation of public and private space. The centre of the city is home of the city's most important civic public spaces, including the *agora* (i.e., the central component of the city, the

© The Author(s) 2019
M. Dovjak and A. Kukec, *Creating Healthy and Sustainable Buildings*, https://doi.org/10.1007/978-3-030-19412-3_1

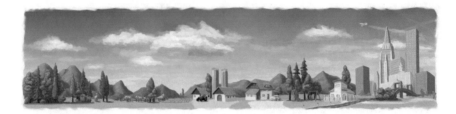

Fig. 1.1 The continuum of space and time of the built environment

marketplace), the *bouleuterion* (i.e., a building that housed the council of citizens in Ancient Greece; an assembly hall), theatres, and temples. Private rooms surround the city's public areas (Glaeser 2011; Boundless 2017).

Although the concept of the built environment is more than 2500 years old, the term emerged in the 1980s and came into widespread use in the 1990s (Crowe 1997).

> McClure and Bartuska (2007, p. 5) described the creative results of human activities throughout history and a holistic and integrated concept of the built environment as: "Everything humanly made, arrange and maintain (e.g., design, plan and build construction), to fulfil human purposes (e.g., needs, wants and values), to mediate the overall environment, with the results affecting the environment in context."

Bartuska (2007) introduced the term "**total built environment**", which is organized into seven interrelated components that emerge from human needs, thoughts, and actions:

- **Products**—include materials and commodities generally created to extend the human capacity to perform specific tasks
- **Interiors**—arranged groupings of products generally enclosed within a structure
- **Structures**—planned groupings of spaces defined by and composed of products
- **Landscapes**—exterior areas and/or settings for planned groupings of spaces and structures
- **Cities**—groupings of structures and landscapes of varying sizes and complexities
- **Regions**—groupings of cities and landscapes of various sizes and complexities
- **Earth**—groupings of regions consisting of cities and landscapes—the entire planet.

In Bartuska's definition, every component of the built environment is defined and shaped by context; each and all of the individual elements contribute either positively or negatively to the overall quality of environments, both built and natural and to human-environment relationships (Bartuska 2007). In the processes related to planning and designing of built environments from micro, medium, to a global scale, the negative consequences of anthropogenic activities (i.e., air, soil, water, food contamination) should be fully prevented. In setting preventive measures, public-awareness and individual responsibility are vital. Although the built environment is distinguished from the natural environment, it should be in harmony with it (Bartuska 2007).

Due to holistic endeavours and the extent of our human-made environment, the term "**built environment**" is used in various disciplines, including architecture, civil engineering, mechanical engineering, occupational safety, and environmental and public health.

> The Construction Industry Council (CIC 2017) suggests that the built environment "encompasses all forms of building (e.g., housing, industrial, commercial, hospitals, schools), and civil engineering infrastructure, both above and below ground and includes the managed landscapes between and around buildings."

In recent years, environmental public health research has expanded the definition of "**built environment**". In environmental public health, built environment refers to physical environments that are designed with health and wellness as integral parts of the communities. The built environment significantly affects the health of individuals and communities. This was most evident during the industrial revolution when infectious diseases were the primary public health threat: unsanitary conditions and overcrowded urban areas facilitated the spread of infection (Perdue et al. 2003).

During the 19th century, the connection between environmental public health and the built environment became increasingly apparent. In this field, dramatic improvements in environmental public health were made possible in industrialized nations through changes in the built environment. The installation of comprehensive sewer systems, improvements in building designs to ensure that residents had light and fresh air, and the movement of residential areas away from noxious industrial facilities all brought significant improvements in health.

Industrialization highlighted the relationship between the built environment and environmental public health (Rosen 1993) which seemed to have diminished in the mid-20th century. Infectious diseases had been brought under control and, as a result, the layout and planning of cities came to be viewed as a matter of aesthetics or economics, but not health (Perdue et al. 2003).

Today, the majority of public health problems are related to chronic diseases. The built environment influences the public's health, particularly in relation to such diseases. However, many urban and suburban environments are not well designed to facilitate healthy behaviour or create the conditions that protect health. Health officials can provide information about healthy living, but if people live in poorly designed physical environments, their health will suffer (Perdue et al. 2003).

A sedentary lifestyle and poor nutrition contribute to obesity, a risk factor for some of the leading causes of mortality, including cardiovascular disease, diabetes, stroke, and some cancers (Mokdad et al. 2003; Glanz et al. 2016).

Although the links between physical activity, proper nutrition, a clean environment, and health are well known, the current built environment does not promote healthy lifestyles. Many urban environments lack safe open spaces that encourage exercise and access to nutritious food and promote the use of alcohol and tobacco products through outdoor advertising (Perdue et al. 2003). A spread-out suburban design facilitates reliance on automobiles, increasing pollution and decreasing the time spent walking. Research has indicated that the way neighbourhoods are planned can affect both the physical activity and mental health of the communities' residents (Renalds et al. 2010; Kent and Thompson 2014). Studies have shown that built environments designed to improve physical activity do, in fact, demonstrate higher rates of physical activity, which in turn positively affects health (Carlson et al. 2012). The environment is integral in promoting physical activity (Goldstein 2002).

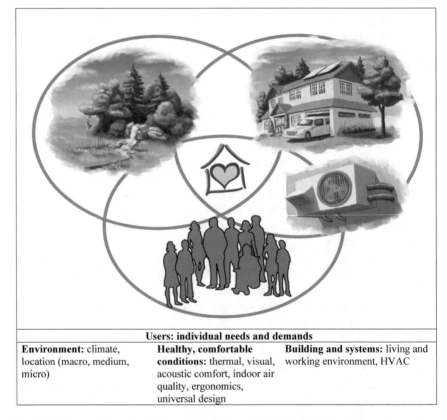

Users: individual needs and demands		
Environment: climate, location (macro, medium, micro)	**Healthy, comfortable conditions:** thermal, visual, acoustic comfort, indoor air quality, ergonomics, universal design	**Building and systems:** living and working environment, HVAC

Fig. 1.2 The cut-off crowd of influencing parameters of the design of the built environment

The built environment affects health in a number of ways. It is not sufficient to educate people regarding healthy lifestyles; the built environment must promote, or at least allow engagement in healthy behaviours. Therefore, it is necessary to take into account all influencing parameters of the design of the built environment (Fig. 1.2). Legislation on the built environment can be used as a tool to accomplish this goal (Gostin 2000).

1.2 A Historical Background of the Built Environment

Vernacular buildings are buildings that are designed based on local needs, availability of construction materials, and reflect local traditions. Vernacular architecture relied on the design skills and tradition of local builders. However, since the late 19th century many professional architects have worked in versions of this style. It tends to evolve to reflect the environmental, cultural, technological, economic, and historical contexts (Scott 1996; Abbacan-Tuguic 2016). Principles of vernacular buildings are incorporated into bioclimatic design processes (Krainer 1993a). Bioclimatic design, based on common sense and location endowments, results in comfortable indoor conditions. Socrates's sun-tempered house and Preskar's cottage, Velika planina, are chosen as examples of bioclimatic designs of vernacular buildings (Figs. 1.3 and 1.4).

Socrates's House or sun-tempered house was designed by Socrates, the Greek philosopher, about 2500 years ago. It is a trapezoid-shaped house with the long side facing the sun. A house with such an ideal shape stays warm in winter and cool in summer without reliance on outside energy sources. The roof overhang on the south blocks the hot summer sun yet allows the winter sun to penetrate the home. The roof slopes down in the back to protect from winter winds (Natural Building Blog 2013).

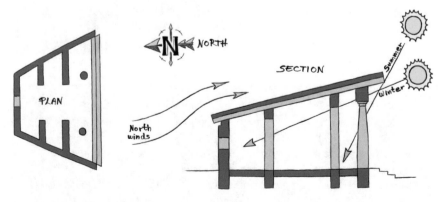

Fig. 1.3 Socrates' sun-tempered house

Fig. 1.4 Reconstructed Preskar's cottage, Velika planina, Slovenia (oval form, square form)

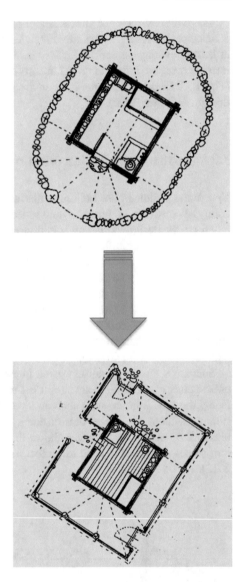

In Book III, Chapter VIII, of Xenophon's Memorabilia of Socrates, written a few decades after Aeschylus, and in the midst of a Greek wood fuel shortage, the Greek philosopher, Socrates, observed: "Now in houses with a south aspect, the sun's rays penetrate into the porticos in winter, but in the summer, the path of the sun is right over our heads and above the roof, so that there is shade. If then this is the best arrangement, we should build the south side loftier to get the winter sun and the north side lower to keep out the winter winds. To put it shortly, the house in which the owner can find a pleasant retreat at all seasons and can store his belongings safely is presumably at once the pleasantest and the most beautiful."

Marcus Vitruvius Pollio (80–70 BC) was a Roman author, architect, civil engineer, and military engineer. He is the author *of De architectura*, known today as *The Ten Books on Architecture*. According to Vitruvius, every architect should focus on three central themes when preparing a design for a building: *firmitas* (strength), *utilitas* (functionality), and *venustas* (beauty). In his work, he explained that the climate determinates the style of the house and how the particular purposes of different rooms require different exposures, suited to convenience and to the quarters of the sky (e.g., winter dining rooms and bathrooms should have a south-western exposure; bedrooms and libraries ought to have an eastern exposure) (Vitruvius Pollio and Morgan 1960).

Another example of vernacular architecture is shepherd housing, found on the high mountain plateau of Velika planina in Slovenia. It demonstrates a bridge between ancient patterns and modern times (Fig. 1.4). The home of a shepherd has a square form, surrounded by oval stable and hay storage, which serves as a buffer zone. The construction follows a kind of double envelope principle. The inside living space is separated from the outside by a zone which was warmed by the metabolic heat of animals or was filled with a material that has unique heat insulation properties. The foundations are made of stone, and the rest of the construction is made of wood (Krainer 1993a). For centuries, the farmers chose the same location to place their Shepard cottages: in areas protected from wind and dampness, entries facing south.

Unfortunately, the settlement was destroyed during the First World War. After the war, the settlement was rebuilt, but only partially respecting the old patterns. The oval forms were replaced by square forms; the roofs were coloured with allegedly protective dark coverings. This has two main negative consequences: firstly, changed the colour climate of the environment (original cottages had the silver-grey colour of aged timber), and secondly, the dark colour has, as opposed to the natural colour of wood, larger solar absorptivity, which causes a higher degree of stretching and shrinkage of wood. All this means the shorter lifetime of wood (Krainer 1993a).

Nowadays, the design of built environments is challenged by various problems related to energy, environment and health, e.g., climate changes, energy security, depletion of natural resources, heat-related mortality and morbidity. The future climate conditions worldwide are projected in the continuation of the increase of (1) temperatures and extreme temperature conditions (extreme cold and hot days); (2) winter and spring precipitation; (3) frequency and intensity of extreme precipitation events, (4) short-term and long-term droughts, (5) heat waves (IPPC 2018; Melillo et al. 2014). Climate change can, therefore, affect human health in two ways: first, by changing the severity or frequency of health problems that are already affected by climate or weather factors; and second, by creating unprecedented or unanticipated health problems or health threats in places where they have not previously occurred. According to USGCRP (2016), the adverse effects of climate change on human health can be divided on: temperature-related death and illness, respiratory and cardiovascular impacts of poor indoor and outdoor air quality, negative impacts of extreme events, vector-borne disease, water-related illness, negative impacts on food safety, nutrition and distribution, negative consequences on mental health and wellbeing. Especially vulnerable to all those changes are children, elderly, and economically disadvantaged groups.

According to climate changes and their problems, building design as a whole or their separate parts must follow the basic principles of bioclimatic design that starts from climate and location dynamic characteristics. While the principles of bioclimatic design coincide with human existence, they are often neglected in current design practice and might result in deteriorated conditions. Current and future construction and renovation must be based on the main goal of bioclimatic building design, i.e., to provide the usage of positive influences on the particular location (i.e., mass, energy, information) together with the protection against negative influences. Accordingly, passive solar elements shall be introduced (e.g., direct gain design, indirect gain design, isolated gain design, shading, night cooling, evaporative cooling, etc.). Sustainable use of locally accessible natural materials for buildings as a whole or their separate parts has to be considered, such as wood (Schickhofer and Hasewend 2000; Kuzman Kitek and Kutnar 2014; Kunič 2016). Technology is only one of the pillars of the design. Such an approach results in healthy and comfortable sustainable built environments.

> It is important to understand its bioclimatic aspect, that is, the relationship between the built environment and us as living systems. This is not only for those involved in building-related profession but also for others, since all of us as living systems spend most of the time within the built environment (Shukuya 2019, p. 2).

1.3 Morphology of Engineering Design of Built Environments

The built environment includes living and working environments, depending on the use of the building and on the activities performed. As is often the case, a living environment is also a working environment and vice versa. For example, a nursing home (i.e., convalescent home, skilled nursing facility, care home, rest home or intermediate care) is a living environment for people who require continual nursing care and have significant difficulty coping with the required activities of daily living (e.g., elderly and younger adults with physical or mental disabilities). For nursing aides and skilled nurses, who are usually available 24 h a day, a nursing home is their working environment (Reinhard et al. 2008).

> The methodology of the design of a healthy built environment was introduced by Krainer (1993b) and has been upgraded.

The starting point of every engineering design process is the definition of the main purpose/s of a building. The **purpose of the building** depends on the building classification type: e.g., commercial buildings, residential buildings, medical buildings, educational buildings, government buildings, industrial buildings, military buildings, parking structures and storage, religious buildings, transport buildings, non-buildings, infrastructure, power providers and others (OJ RS, No. 37/2018). All classified building types have subtypes (National Institute of Building Sciences 2017). For example, subtypes of medical buildings are hospitals, nursing homes, quarantines and asylums (National Institute of Building Sciences 2017). If we design a nursing home, which is a subtype of a medical building, its design process differs from the design process of a school (educational building type) or office (commercial building type).

Furthermore, more effort should be invested at the beginning of the design process when designing **multipurpose buildings** with various activities (i.e., office/residential building, office/commercial building; healthcare service/office/residential building). The definition of a building's purpose and activity in the building impacts all steps of engineering design.

After the definition of the purpose of the building, the characteristic of a specific location should be taken into consideration. It often happens that a building is planned without knowing the **bioclimatic endowment** of the specific location. Moreover, building plans are often transferred from one location to another, without taking into account bioclimatic design approaches. This leads to an energy, environmentally, and functionally inadequate built environment with unhealthy and uncomfortable living and working conditions.

The main characteristics of bioclimatic endowment cover:

- **Topographic, geographical features, geomorphology**
- **Climate type/subtype, climate changes, meteorological conditions**
- **Biotic diversity, flora, fauna**
- **Sources and quality of water, soil, air and food, history of pollution**
- **Social determinants (cultural creativity, religion, etc.)**
- **Others**.

Listed characteristics of the bioclimatic endowment may present strengths or weaknesses for the design process depending on timescale and space. For example, renewable energy sources available at the specific location (i.e., sunlight, wind, rain, tides, waves, and geothermal heat) could provide energy for building operation, which is a major advantage in bioclimatic design (Stritih and Koželj 2017). Furthermore, Directive 2009/28/EC sets a binding target that by 2020, 20% of energy consumption must come from renewable sources. In contrast, seasonal temperature variations resulting in overcooling and overheating represent a disadvantage in bioclimatic design. Therefore, it is necessary to prevent thermal losses in winter and heat gains in summer with efficient building envelope systems (Hudobivnik et al. 2016; Pajek et al. 2017; Kunič 2017). Defined strengths and weaknesses are stimuli for building envelope design (Krainer 1993b). In addition to the bioclimatic endorsement, **cultural heritage criteria** must also be included in the design. Blecich et al. (2016) highlighted the role of responsible and careful planning for the preservation of cultural heritage buildings to coincide with the application of energy efficiency measures.

At the stage of positioning the building on the specific location, it is important to find optimal orientation and position of **active spaces** inside a building plan (Fig. 1.5).

Fig. 1.5 Schematic of the morphology of engineering design (Krainer 1993b)

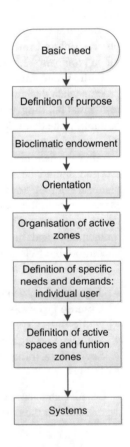

For the optimal position of active spaces inside a building plan, all **activities, requirements, and conditions** for the surrounding active spaces should be taken into consideration in both the indoor and outdoor environments. Particular attention should be dedicated to:

- **Temperature zones** (i.e., group of active spaces with room air temperature difference less than 4 K)
- **Noisy, active spaces** (e.g., machine room, elevator duct, music classroom, garage, laundry room) and **quiet, noise-protected active spaces** (e.g., patient room, library, bedroom)
- **Spaces with special requirements and clean spaces** (e.g., obstetric bedroom unit for new-borns, intensive therapy, sterile spaces such as operating theatre, neonatology, isolation rooms)
- **Spaces without special requirements** (e.g., halls, administrative facilities, service; unclean spaces, e.g., waiting room, laundry, toilets, corridors).

The positioning of active spaces inside a building plan has an impact on other performed activities (i.e., cleaning, disinfection, and maintenance), installation of HVAC (heating, ventilating and air conditioning) systems and air quality issues (i.e., classes of indoor air quality).

Since the built environment is manifested in physical objects and places (Bartuska 2007), it is necessary to define **active spaces** and **functional zones**.

BOX 1.1 Active space

Active space is a space in the built environment that can be positioned in inside or outside environments. It is a three-dimensional space intended for specific activities circumscribed by constructional complexes. Active space is characterized by specific volume, demands and needs, according to the purpose and performed activities (e.g., kitchen or dining room in a residential building; patient room or a treatment room in a hospital).

BOX 1.2 Active zone

User zone inside active space; a space or a group of spaces within a building with any combination of heating, cooling or lighting requirements sufficiently similar so that desired conditions can be maintained by a single controlling device (ISO/TC 205/WG 002: 1998). Definition of active zones and active spaces presents one of the initial steps of the engineering design process. Based on the defined active zones and spaces together with user characteristics and their needs and demands, the required and/or recommended indoor environmental conditions are determined that have to be created by effective systems. Circumvention of the first steps of design often results in uncomfortable or unhealthy conditions.

> **BOX 1.3 Functional zone**
> The physical limits of active space present functional zones. The functional zone is a boundary interface that demarcates active spaces and physically presents constructional complex. All functional zones have specific functions that determine the composition and used materials (e.g., exterior wall, roof, floor). Optimal composition of constructional complexes (i.e., exterior, interior elements) has a beneficiary effect on the user-building-system performance relationship.

Examples of functional zones and their characteristic functions are:

- The functional zone between two temperature zones has to be **thermally insulated**
- The functional zone between spaces without special requirements/unclean/clean/sterile active spaces needs **final coating material** resistant to cleaning and disinfection, special material selection and execution
- The functional zone between noisy, active spaces (e.g., machine room, elevator duct, music classroom, garage, laundry room) in quiet and noise-protected active spaces (e.g., patient room, library, bedroom) needs proper **sound insulation** against airborne noise, structure-borne noise and room acoustics
- The functional zone between wet or humid active spaces needs a **water-proofing system, a damp-proof membrane**.

The composition of functional zones and selection of materials depends on demands and conditions for active space. Demands and conditions are defined by national and international regulations, standards, and recommendations. There are various demands and conditions, such as sanitary-technical, hygienic, microbiologic, aseptic, fire safety and air quality (Table 1.1).

Table 1.1 Diversity of requirements and needs in the design process of the built environment (TSG-12640-001: 2008; CPR 305/2011)

Basic requirementsfor construction works	Specific requirements for active spaces
• Hygiene, health and the environment • Mechanical resistance and stability • Safety in case of fire • Safety and accessibility in use • Protection against noise • Energy economy and heat retention • Sustainable use of natural resources • Protection of cultural heritage • Others	• Health and occupational safety procedures • Parameters of overall comfort conditions (thermal comfort, daylight, acoustics, air quality) • Hygienic conditions (cleaning, maintenance, used materials in spaces without special requirements/unclean/clean/sterile active spaces) • Mechanical properties (e.g., wear of floor, which is defined by the load or the frequency and gravity of traffic in each active space) • Requirements relating to the material properties and execution • Chemical properties (i.e., zero emission materials, nontoxic materials) • Environmental safety • Safety against electromagnetic radiation • Ergonomics • Universal design • Others

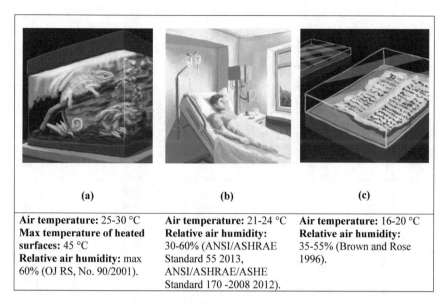

(a)	(b)	(c)
Air temperature: 25-30 °C **Max temperature of heated surfaces:** 45 °C **Relative air humidity:** max 60% (OJ RS, No. 90/2001).	**Air temperature:** 21-24 °C **Relative air humidity:** 30-60% (ANSI/ASHRAE Standard 55 2013, ANSI/ASHRAE/ASHE Standard 170 -2008 2012).	**Air temperature:** 16-20 °C **Relative air humidity:** 35-55% (Brown and Rose 1996).

Fig. 1.6 Examples of active spaces with individualized microclimate conditions: **a** iguana in active space, **b** patient room in hospital, **c** museum artefact

An important step is to define a complete list of all **specific demands and conditions** for active spaces. The main guidance is the **intended use** (e.g., play-room in kindergarten, patient room in a hospital, living room in a nursing home, museum), **target users** (e.g., children, patients, elderly, reptiles, tropical plants) and **goods** (e.g., artefacts, food) (Fig. 1.6).

In Table 1.2 selected examples of temperature requirements for various building types, active spaces, and target users are presented. As indicated, the requirements for active spaces differ between built environment types, active spaces, and target users. When designers of built environments are creating a list of specific requirements, it is important to include all relevant information from:

- **Requirements, recommendations**
- **Scientific studies**
- **Expert knowledge, and**
- **User opinion**.

Specifically, current requirements and recommendations are often defined on the characteristics of average users and not vulnerable ones. For example, temperature requirements and recommendations for a playground in a kindergarten may result in uncomfortable conditions for children (recommended operative temperature ranges for winter and summer periods, different categories).

Additionally, in built environments, it is often necessary to simultaneously achieve the requirements for two different user types in the same active space. For example, in a patient room for burnt patients, user-centred healing-oriented

Table 1.2 Selection of temperature requirements according to building type, active space and target user

Built environment type	Active space, target users	Required/recommended value	Sources
Living environment: residential buildings	Living spaces, residents	• Required air temperature for a seated person in the occupied zone during the non-heating period is 22–26 °C (preferably 23–25 °C), during heating period is 19–24 °C (preferably 20–22 °C) • Required floor surface temperature is 17–26° C, in the case of floor heating up to 29 ° C; prevented local radiative asymmetry • Required relative air humidity below 60%, which reduces the growth of microorganisms • Required optimum operative temperature depending on the metabolic rate and effective clothing insulation	• OJ RS, No. 42/2002, chang. • OJ RS, No. 73/2000, chang. • CR 1752 (1998) • ISO 7730 (2005) • OJ RS, No. 89/1999, chang. • CSIP (2014) • Brown and Rose (1996) • ANSI/ASHRAE/ASHE Standard 170-2008 (2012) • ASHRAE Handbook (2007) • Maynard and Hochmuth (2007) • OJ RS, No. 90/2001 • EN 15251 (2007) • BS 5454 (2000) • Trček Pečjak and Ivanišin (2017)
Childcare institutions: kindergartens	Playrooms, children	• Active spaces for children must be uniformly heated as follows: at 20 °C in rooms for children, at 23 °C in the rooms for child care up to 3 years, at 18–19° C in sport playroom • The required designed operative temperature for summer is 23.5 °C ± 2.5, for winter is 20.0 °C ± 3.5 • Recommended design criteria for operative temperature for summer period is 23.5 °C ± 1.0 (category A); 23.5 °C ± 2.0 (category B); 23.5 °C ± 2.5 (category C) and for winter period 20.0 °C ± 1.0 (category A); 20.0 °C ± 2.5 (category B); 20.0 °C ± 3.5 (category C) • Recommended operative temperature for summer period is 23.5 °C ± 1.0 (category A); 23.5 °C ± 2.0 (category B); 23.5 °C ± 2.5 (category C) and for winter period is 20.0 °C ± 1.0 (category A); 22.0 °C ± 2.5 (category B); 22.0 °C ± 3.5 (category C) • Recommended minimal design values of operative temperature for heating (winter season, 1 clo, clothing insulation) is 19.0 °C for Category I; 17.5 °C for Category II; 16.5 °C for Category III	• OJ RS, No. 42/2002, chang. • OJ RS, No. 73/2000, chang. • CR 1752 (1998) • ISO 7730 (2005) • OJ RS, No. 89/1999, chang. • CSIP (2014) • Brown and Rose (1996) • ANSI/ASHRAE/ASHE Standard 170-2008 (2012) • ASHRAE Handbook (2007) • Maynard and Hochmuth (2007) • OJ RS, No. 90/2001 • EN 15251 (2007) • BS 5454 (2000) • Trček Pečjak and Ivanišin (2017)

(continued)

Table 1.2 (continued)

Built environment type	Active space, target users	Required/recommended value	Sources
		• Recommended maximal design values of operative temperature for cooling (summer season, 0.5 clo) is 24.5 °C for Category I; 25.5 °C for Category II; 26.0 °C for Category III • Required relative air humidity in the rooms for children is 40–60%	
Working environment: offices	Staff	• Air temperature in the working areas during working hours has to take into account physiological needs of workers, the nature of work, and the physical load of workers, with the exception of work in cold rooms • Air temperature in the working areas should not exceed +28 °C. The exceptions are hot workplaces, where the air temperature may exceed +28 °C; however, the employer must ensure that air temperature in service areas, hallways and stairs is not higher than +20 °C • Required air temperature for a seated person in the occupied zone during the non-heating period is 22–26 °C (preferably 23–25 °C), during heating period is 19–24 °C (preferably 20–22 °C) • The floor surface temperature of the working areas should not be less than 19 °C and not higher than 29 °C. Floor surface temperature of the working areas in which the workers spend more than 2 h per day, may not be higher than the maximum 27 °C • Required designed operative temperature for summer period is 24.5 °C ± 2.5, for winter period is 22.0 °C ± 3.0 • Recommended design criteria for operative temperature for summer period is 24.5 °C ± 1.0 (category A); 24.5 °C ± 1.5 (category B); 24.5 °C ± 2.5 (category C) and for winter period is 22.0 °C ± 1.0 (category A); 22.0 °C ± 2.0 (category B); 22.0 °C ± 3.0 (category C) • Recommended operative temperature for summer period is 24.5 °C ± 1.0 (category A); 24.5 °C ± 1.5 (category B); 24.5 °C ± 2.5 (category C) and for winter period is 22.0 °C ± 1.0 (category A); 22.0 °C ± 2.0 (category B); 22.0 °C ± 3.0 (category C) • Recommended minimal design values of operative temperature for heating (winter season, 1 clo) is 21.0 °C for Category I; 20.0 °C for Category II; 19.0 °C for Category III	• OJ RS, No. 42/2002, chang. • OJ RS, No. 73/2000, chang. • CR 1752 (1998) • ISO 7730 (2005) • OJ RS, No. 89/1999, chang. • CSIP (2014) • Brown and Rose (1996) • ANSI/ASHRAE/ASHE Standard 170-2008 (2012) • ASHRAE Handbook (2007) • Maynard and Hochmuth (2007) • OJ RS, No. 90/2001 • EN 15251 (2007) • BS 5454 (2000) • Trček Pečjak and Ivanišin (2017)

(continued)

Table 1.2 (continued)

Built environment type	Active space, target users	Required/recommended value	Sources
		• Recommended maximal design values of operative temperature for cooling (summer season, 0.5 clo) is 25.5 °C for Category I; 26.0 °C for Category II; 27.0 °C for Category III • Relative humidity of supplied air depends on its temperature and may not exceed the following values: 80% at room air temperature $T_{ai} \geq 20$ °C; 73% at $T_{ai} \geq 22$ °C; 65% at $T_{ai} \geq 24$ °C; 60% at $T_{ai} \geq 26$ °C; 55% at $T_{ai} \geq 28$ °C • Relative humidity of the inlet air must not be lower than 30%	
Cultural institutions: museums	Artefacts	• Recommended air temperature and relative air humidity in cabinets for palaeontological, geological, mineralogical collections; botanical, entomological, zoological materials: 40–50%, 16–20 °C • Recommended air temperature and relative air humidity for open spaces in storage areas: 35–55%, 16–20 °C • Open storage areas where large materials are stored (e.g., petrological, large taxidermy): relative humidity 35–60%, air temperature 16–23 °C • Stability of the humidity control is far more important than the precise level. Relative air humidity of between 45–55% with daily fluctuations held to ±5% relative air humidity • Conservation and exhibition of canvas paintings: relative air humidity 50–60% (± 2.5%), air temperature 18–22 °C (standard deviation of monthly measurements of air temperature and relative air humidity should not exceed 1) • Recommendations for storage and exhibition of archival documents: bound material —paper: air temperature 13–18 °C, relative air humidity 55–65%; non-bound material—paper: air temperature 13–18 °C, relative air humidity 40%; other materials, except paper and parchment: air temperature 13–16 °C, relative air humidity 50–60%	• OJ RS, No. 42/2002, chang. • OJ RS, No. 73/2000, chang. • CR 1752 (1998) • ISO 7730 (2005) • OJ RS, No. 89/1999, chang. • CSIP (2014) • Brown and Rose (1996) • ANSI/ASHRAE/ASHE Standard 170-2008 (2012) • ASHRAE Handbook (2007) • Maynard and Hochmuth (2007) • OJ RS, No. 90/2001 • EN 15251 (2007) • BS 5454 (2000) • Trček Pečjak and Ivanišin (2017)
Health institutions: hospital ward	Patients	• Requirement depends on the health status, hygienic requirements, activity • Recommended air temperature ranges from 20 °C to 26 °C due to the specifics of the type of ward facility • A ward for severe burn injuries should have temperature controls that permit adjusting the room temperature up to 32 °C and relative humidity up to 95%	• OJ RS, No. 42/2002, chang. • OJ RS, No. 73/2000, chang. • CR 1752 (1998) • ISO 7730 (2005) • OJ RS, No. 89/1999, chang. • CSIP (2014)

Table 1.2 (continued)

Built environment type	Active space, target users	Required/recommended value	Sources
		• The operative environmental temperature needed to provide thermal neutrality for healthy baby nursed naked in draft-free surroundings of uniform temperature, and moderate humidity after birth is in the range from 35 °C (for 1 kg birth weight) to 32 °C (more than 2.5 kg of birth weight)	• Brown and Rose (1996) • ANSI/ASHRAE/ASHE Standard 170-2008 (2012) • ASHRAE Handbook (2007) • Maynard and Hochmuth (2007) • OJ RS, No. 90/2001 • EN 15251 (2007) • BS 5454 (2000) • Trček Pečjak and Ivanišin (2017)
Health institutions: hospital wards	Operating rooms for specialized procedures	• Temperature requirements for operating rooms for specialized procedures for cardiac surgery at 17 °C, for corneal surgery at 18–24 °C, and for paediatric surgeries at 30 °C	• OJ RS, No. 42/2002, chang. • OJ RS, No. 73/2000, chang. • CR 1752 (1998) • ISO 7730 (2005) • OJ RS, No. 89/1999, chang. • CSIP (2014) • Brown and Rose (1996) • ANSI/ASHRAE/ASHE Standard 170-2008 (2012) • ASHRAE Handbook (2007) • Maynard and Hochmuth (2007) • OJ RS, No. 90/2001 • EN 15251 (2007) • BS 5454 (2000) • Trček Pečjak and Ivanišin (2017)
Food facility: storing food	Vegetables	• Recommended air temperature and relative humidity depends on hygienic demands for food storage (food safety, HACCP) • Recommended air temperature and relative humidity: 0–1.7 °C, 95-98% for beets, carrots, parsnips, radish, rutabaga, turnips, yacon; 0–1.7 °C, 90–95% for celery, cabbage; 0–1.7 °C, 18.3–23.9 °C, 50–75% for garlic, onions; 3.3–4.5 °C, 80–90% for potatoes,	• OJ RS, No. 42/2002, chang. • OJ RS, No. 73/2000, chang. • CR 1752 (1998) • ISO 7730 (2005) • OJ RS, No. 89/1999, chang. • CSIP (2014)

(continued)

Table 1.2 (continued)

Built environment type	Active space, target users	Required/recommended value	Sources
		10.0–15.6 °C, 50–75% for pumpkins; 10.0–15.6 °C, 50–95% for squash, winter; 0–1.7 °C, 95–98% for turnips	• Brown and Rose (1996) • ANSI/ASHRAE/ASHE Standard 170-2008 (2012) • ASHRAE Handbook (2007) • Maynard and Hochmuth (2007) • OJ RS. No. 90/2001 • EN 15251 (2007) • BS 5454 (2000) • Trček Pečjak and Ivanišin (2017)
Zoological facilities: living space	Animals	• Primates: 20–25 °C for maki, 18–25 °C for lemur, 16 °C for a chimpanzee • Rodentia: 15 °C for a capybara • Carnivora: 18 °C for a wildcat, $\geq$ 15 °C for tiger, lion • Perissodactyla: 18 °C for a rhinoceros • Artiodactyla: 15 °C for a giraffe • Passeriformes, tropical bird: >10 °C; • Parrots: >10 °C • Lizards (Sauria): *Iguana*: 35–30 °C of air temperature, 45 °C of max temperature of heated surfaces; *Dipsosaurus*: 25–30 °C of air temperature, 50 °C of max temperature of heated surfaces; *Corytophanes* 20–28 °C of air temperature, 35 °C of max temperature of heated surfaces • Chameleons (Chamaeleonidae): *Calaumma gallus* 32 °C for radiative heat, 60% relative air humidity • Snakes (Serpents): Typhlops: 26–30 °C of air temperature during the day, slightly cooler during the night, 28–33 °C of local max temperature for types of dry habitats	• OJ RS, No. 42/2002, chang. • OJ RS, No. 73/2000, chang. • CR 1752 (1998) • ISO 7730 (2005) • OJ RS, No. 89/1999, chang. • CSIP (2014) • Brown and Rose (1996) • ANSI/ASHRAE/ASHE Standard 170-2008 (2012) • ASHRAE Handbook (2007) • Maynard and Hochmuth (2007) • OJ RS, No. 90/2001 • EN 15251 (2007) • BS 5454 (2000) • Trček Pečjak and Ivanišin (2017)

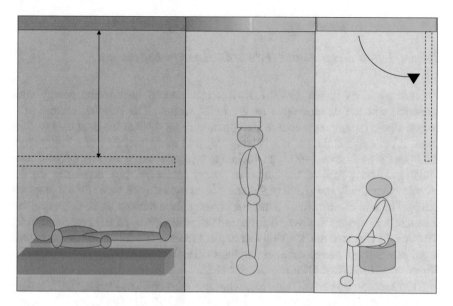

Fig. 1.7 Individualization of active space in a hospital environment (Dovjak 2012, p. 147)

conditions for patients and comfort conditions for staff should be created (Dovjak 2012; Dovjak et al. 2013, 2014, 2018). Nowadays systems are designed that enable the individualization of active space (i.e., innovative systems to achieve healthy, comfortable, and stimulating conditions for individual users) (Fig. 1.7).

The requirements for the parameters of thermal comfort depend on the intended use of the building, the type of the active space, the activity, and the characteristics of the individual users (e.g., people, animals, plants). All listed requirements present input data for the design of the building. By considering them, designers will follow the morphology of the engineering design process. Among the last steps is the selection and installation of efficient HVAC systems that support the functionality of the whole building.

> **The purpose is to design a healthy, comfortable building (i.e., residential, public) with minimal possible use of energy and environmental impacts. Health, wellbeing and comfort are the core of the whole process of design. For this purpose, our starting point is individual vulnerable user with specific needs and demands (Dovjak et al. 2018).**

1.4   Legal Framework

1.4.1   Legal Framework Towards Energy Efficiency

The energy crisis in the 1970s led to greater interest in reducing energy consumption and use of renewable energy in all sectors. The building sector is the largest single energy consumer in Europe, absorbing 40% of the final energy. The stock of buildings in the EU is relatively old, with more than 40% of it built before 1960 and 90% before 1990. Old buildings typically use more energy than new buildings. About 75% of buildings are energy inefficient and, depending on the Member State, only 0.4–1.2% of the stock is renovated each year (EPBD proposal 2016). The rate at which new buildings either replace this old stock or expand the total stock, is about 1% a year (European Parliament 2016; EPBD proposal 2016). The situation leads to the adoption and implementation of national and international legislation toward energy efficient buildings (EPBD-r 2010/31/EU; CPR 305/2011; Directive 2012/27/EU; Directive 2009/28/EC).

The European Union (EU) aims to achieve an energy efficiency target of 20% energy savings by 2020 (EC 2020) and 27% by 2030 (EC 2030). The Energy Efficiency Directive 2012/27/EU (Directive 2012/27/EU) and the Energy Performance of Buildings Directive (EPBD-r 2010/31/EU) are the main energy efficiency policy instruments in the European Union for reaching these goals. Member States respond to the EED through national action plans (EPA 2017a).

The Directive 2012/27/EU is a European Union directive which mandates energy efficiency improvements within the European Union, and it introduces legally binding measures to encourage efforts to use energy more efficiently in all stages and sectors of the supply chain. It establishes a common framework for the promotion of energy efficiency within the EU in order to meet its energy efficiency headline target of 20% by 2020. The EPBD-r 2010/31/EU is an EU directive on Energy Performance of Buildings and sets the so-called "20-20-20" goals: 20% increase in energy efficiency, 20% reduction of CO_2 emissions, and 20% renewables by 2020. The Renewable Energy Directive 2009/28/EC (Directive 2009/28/EC) mandates levels of renewable energy use within the European Union. The directive requires that 20% of the energy consumed within the European Union be renewable. This target is pooled among the member states. Overall the potential to achieve energy savings is the highest in the residential sector, which accounts for 40% of the EU's final energy consumption and 36% of its greenhouse gas emissions (Climate policy info hub 2017). On 30 November 2016, the Commission proposed an update of the EPBD. The main objectives of the EPBD proposal (2016) are: integrating long-term building renovation strategies, supporting the mobilization of financing and creating a clear vision for a decarbonized building stock by 2050; encouraging the use of information and communication technology and smart technologies to ensure that buildings operate efficiently; and streamlining provisions where they have not delivered the expected results. On 19 June 2018, the revised Energy Performance of Buildings Directive (EU) 2018/844 was published in the Official Journal of the European Union, following its formal approval by the Parliament on 17 April 2018 and by the Council of Ministers on 14 May 2018. The directive came into effect on 9 July 2018.

Construction Products Regulation, No. 305/2011 (CPR 305/2011) is an umbrella legal act on construction products.

BOX 1.4 Construction product

'Construction product' means any product or kit that is produced and placed on the market for incorporation in a permanent manner in construction works or parts thereof and the performance of which has an effect on the performance of the construction works with respect to the basic requirements for construction works (CPR 305/2011).

CPR is designed to simplify and clarify the existing framework for the placing on the market of construction products. Provisions of the CPR seek to:

- Clarify the affixing of CE marking to construction products. Introduce the need to issue a declaration of performance as a basis for CE marking
- Define clear rules for the assessment and verification of constancy-of-performance (AVCP) systems applicable to construction products (former Attestation of Conformity AoC)
- Define the role and responsibilities of manufacturers, distributors, importers, notified bodies, technical assessment bodies, market surveillance and Member States' authorities as regards the application of this EU regulation. Introduce simplified procedures enabling cost reductions for businesses, especially SMEs (small and medium-sized enterprises)
- Provide a clear framework for the harmonized technical specifications (i.e., harmonized standards and European Assessment Documents) (CPR 305/2011).

BOX 1.5 Construction works

'Construction works' means buildings and civil engineering works (CPR 305/2011). All subjects that are involved in the building design process must be aware that construction works and construction products must satisfy all basic requirements during the whole lifecycle. In this process, Basic Requirement No. 3, Hygiene, health and the environment, must not be overlooked.

Construction works as a whole and their separate parts must be fit for intended use, taking into account, in particular, the health and safety of users involved throughout the life cycle of the work. Construction works must satisfy the basic requirements for an economically reasonable working life (Table 1.3). All

Table 1.3 Basic requirements for construction works in the field of built environment (CPR 305/2011)

Basic requirement	Description
1. Mechanical resistance and stability	The construction works must be designed and built in such a way that the loadings that are liable to act on them during their construction and use will not lead to any of the following: (a) collapse of the whole or part of the work; (b) major deformations to an inadmissible degree; (c) damage to other parts of the construction works or to fittings or installed equipment as a result of major deformation of the load-bearing construction; (d) damage by an event to an extent disproportionate to the original cause
2. Safety in case of fire	The construction works must be designed and built in such a way that in the event of an outbreak of fire: (a) the load-bearing capacity of the construction can be assumed for a specific period; (b) the generation and spread of fire and smoke within the construction works are limited; (c) the spread of fire to neighbouring construction works is limited; (d) occupants can leave the construction works or be rescued by other means; (e) the safety of rescue teams is taken into consideration
3. Hygiene, health, and the environment	The construction works must be designed and built in such a way that they will, throughout their life cycle, not be a threat to the hygiene or health and safety of workers, occupants, or neighbours, nor have an exceedingly high impact, over their entire life cycle, on the environmental quality or on the climate during their construction, use, and demolition, in particular as a result of any of the following: (a) the giving-off of toxic gas; (b) the emissions of dangerous substances, volatile organic compounds (VOC), greenhouse gases or dangerous particles into indoor or outdoor air; (c) the emission of dangerous radiation; (d) the release of dangerous substances into ground water, marine waters, surface waters or soil; (e) the release of dangerous substances into drinking water or substances that have an otherwise negative impact on drinking water; (f) faulty discharge of waste water, emission of flue gases or faulty disposal of solid or liquid waste; (g) dampness in parts of the construction works or on surfaces within the construction works
4. Safety and accessibility in use	The construction works must be designed and built in such a way that they do not present unacceptable risks of accidents or damage in service or in operation, such as slipping, falling, collision, burns, electrocution, injury from explosion and burglaries. In particular, construction works must be designed and built taking into consideration accessibility and use for disabled persons
5. Protection against noise	The construction works must be designed and built in such a way that noise perceived by the occupants or people nearby is kept to a level that will not threaten their health and will allow them to sleep, rest, and work in satisfactory conditions

(continued)

Table 1.3 (continued)

Basic requirement	Description
6. Energy economy and heat retention	The construction works and their heating, cooling, lighting, and ventilation equipment must be designed and built in such a way that the amount of energy they require in use shall be low when the account is taken of the occupants and of the climatic conditions of the location. Construction works must also be energy-efficient, using as little energy as possible during their construction and dismantling
7. Sustainable use of natural resources	The construction works must be designed, built, and demolished in such a way that the use of natural resources is sustainable and in particular ensure the following: (a) reuse or recyclability of the construction works, their materials and parts after demolition; (b) durability of the construction works; (c) use of environmentally compatible raw and secondary materials in the construction works

requirements are transferred and implemented in the national legislation (e.g. Building Act OJ RS, No. 61/2017, chang.).

Buildings are responsible for 40% of energy consumption and 36% of CO_2 emissions in the EU (EC 2016, 2017). While new buildings generally need fewer than three to five litres of heating oil per square metre per year, older buildings consume about 25 litres on average. Some buildings even require up to 60 litres. Currently, about 35% of the EU's buildings are over 50 years old. By improving the energy efficiency of buildings, we could reduce total EU energy consumption by 5–6% and lower CO_2 emissions by about 5% (EC 2017).

Minimizing the environmental impact of buildings (Directive 2009/125/EC; Directive 2009/28/EC; Roadmap 2050; ECF 2010) and improving their energy efficiency (EPBD-r 2010/31/EU; Directive 2012/27/EU) are crucial in achieving the goals set by the Paris Agreement (EC 2017). At the Paris Climate Conference (COP21) in December 2015, 195 countries adopted the first-ever universal, legally binding global climate deal. The agreement sets out a global action plan to put the world on track to avoid dangerous climate change. Governments agreed on a long-term goal of keeping the average warming below 2 °C above pre-industrial levels; to aim to limit the increase to 1.5 °C, since this would significantly reduce the risks and impacts of climate change; on the need for global emissions to peak as soon as possible, recognising that this will take longer for developing countries; to undertake rapid reductions thereafter in accordance with the best available science. The Ecodesign Directive (2009/125/EC) sets minimum efficiency standards for technologies used in the building sector (e.g., boilers, hot water generators, pumps, ventilation, lighting, etc.). The Energy Labelling Directive (Council Directive 92/75/EEC) obliges Member Stats to use energy efficiency labelling schemes for a number of products used in the building sector.

The term "nearly zero-energy building" refers to a building that has a very high energy performance (EPBD). The nearly zero or very low amount of energy that these buildings require should be obtained, to a large extent, from renewable sources, including energy from renewable sources produced on-site or nearby. Member States shall ensure that by 31 December 2020, all new buildings are nearly zero-energy buildings and after 31 December 2018, new buildings occupied and owned by public authorities are nearly zero-energy buildings (EPBD).

The 2030 climate and energy framework sets three key targets for the year 2030: at least 40% cut in greenhouse gas emissions (compared to 1990 levels); at least 27% share of renewable energy; at least 27% improvement in energy efficiency. The framework was adopted by EU leaders in October 2014. It builds on the 2020 climate and energy package. It is also in line with the longer term perspective set out in the Roadmap for moving to a competitive low carbon economy in 2050, the Energy Roadmap 2050 and the Transport White Paper.

An analysis of residential building regulations in eight Member States (BPIE 2015) concludes:

> Indoor health and comfort aspects should be considered to a greater extent in European building codes than is current practice. When planning new nearly zero-energy buildings or nearly zero-energy buildings, refurbishments, requirements for a healthy and pleasant indoor environment should be included (BPIE 2015, p. 10).

1.4.2 Legal Framework Towards a Healthy Environment

The environment is a major determinant of health (WHO 2017). The absence and/or mastering of the risk factors in living and working environments is a basic pre-condition for protecting users' health. Planners and designers of built environments are both legally and morally responsible for designing healthy and comfortable conditions. Furthermore, health is a basic human right and a priority in international and national legal acts and strategic documents. One international legal act that sets out human rights and freedoms and establishes a supervisory mechanism guaranteeing their respect by the Member States is the 29th European Social Charter (OJ RS, No. 24/1999 with changes). Health is one of the basic rights set out in the Charter. Article 11 defines the right to protection of health. With a view to ensuring the effective exercise of the right to health protection, the Parties undertake, either directly or in co-operation with public or private organizations, to take appropriate measures designed, *inter alia*, to remove to the greatest extent possible the causes of ill-health. The European Convention on Human Rights (ECHR) (formally the Convention for the Protection of Human Rights and Fundamental Freedoms) is an international treaty to protect human rights and fundamental freedoms in Europe.

The health and safety of working environments are regulated by the Occupational Safety and Health Convention, 1981, which provides for the adoption of a coherent national occupational safety and health policy, as well as action to be taken by governments and within enterprises to promote occupational safety and health and to improve working conditions. For instance, protection against specific risks is regulated by the Working Environment (Air Pollution, Noise and Vibration) Convention, 1977 (No. 148)—[ratifications]. The convention provides that, to the greatest extent possible, the working environment shall be kept free from any hazards due to air pollution, noise, or vibration. To achieve this, technical measures shall be applied to enterprises or processes, and where this is not possible, supplementary measures regarding the organization of work shall be taken instead. Directive 89/391/EEC - OSH "Framework Directive" aims to introduce measures to encourage improvements in the safety and health of workers. It applies to all sectors of activity, both public and private, except for specific public service activities, such as the armed forces, the police or certain civil protection services.

International legal requirements are transferred and implemented in the national legislation. The fundamental law of the Republic of Slovenia is the Constitution of the Republic of Slovenia. Article 72 stipulates that everyone has the right to a healthy living environment in accordance with the law (Constitution RS).

Many areas are not yet regulated by law and are governed only by recommendations set by different organizations. Regulation and control vary greatly between countries and types of buildings. Regulatory frameworks and standards are influenced by a number of factors (e.g., climatic, cultural, constitutional, economic, and political). For example, England has adopted a qualitative, hazard-based assessment approach for conditions in houses: the Housing Health and Safety Rating System (HHSRS). The system estimates potential threats from the conditions in houses based on 29 potential hazards. The focus of regulations in seven countries can be directed toward five controlling points (i.e., environment and neighbourhood, materials used in construction, design and layout of the dwelling, provided amenities, basic equipment, use and maintenance of the dwelling). Existing housing stock should be improved, and any problems or hazards should be reduced; when the modern quantitative guidelines cannot be met, the approach should focus on the qualitative assessment of the dwelling.

In summary, it is concluded that housing quality (e.g., construction materials, equipment installed, dwelling design) has a major direct or indirect impact on human health and that the health sector and relevant ministries should design and implement more detailed and clear regulations to control housing conditions regarding country priorities and specificities. A good regulatory system is necessary to achieve better health conditions in built environments. There should also be more promotion of health and healthy environments. In the development of housing and health policies, it is also important to consider social aspects (e.g., those on low incomes should be addressed as a priority) and vulnerable members of society (WHO 2017).

Health, comfort and wellbeing are highlighted in EPBD-r 2010/31/EU, EPBD proposal (2016) and Directive (EU) 2018/844:

Measures to improve further the energy performance of buildings should take into account climatic and local conditions as well as indoor climate environment and cost-effectiveness. These measures should not affect other requirements concerning buildings such as accessibility, safety and the intended use of the building (EPBD-r 2010/31/EU, p. 2).

Better performing buildings provide higher comfort levels and wellbeing for their occupants and improve health by reducing mortality and morbidity from a poor indoor climate. Adequately heated and ventilated dwellings alleviate negative health impacts caused by dampness, particularly amongst vulnerable groups such as children and the elderly and those with pre-existing illnesses (EPBD proposal 2016, p. 2).

Member States should support energy performance upgrades of existing buildings that contribute to achieving a healthy indoor environment, … (Directive (EU) 2018/844, p. 3).

1.5 Relevant Problems in the Built Environment, User Complaints

Implementation of legal requirements into national legislation has resulted in shifts towards energy efficiency in the building sector. Measures, such as additional thermal insulation of facades, improved windows, increased air tightness of building envelopes (resistance of the building envelope to inward or outward air leakage), were undertaken in public as well as residential buildings. However, the scope of solutions remains narrow and one-sided. This has resulted in improved energy efficiency, but at the same time in inadequate living and working conditions. Users, experts, and the media have already given attention to this problem.

In 2008, Professor Aleš Krainer of the Faculty of Civil and Geodetic Engineering, Chair of Buildings and Constructional Complexes first drew attention to the so-called passive house movement. In the work titled "Passivhaus contra bioclimatic design" (2008) he compared bioclimatic houses and passive houses in terms of energy and indoor quality parameters. The main guidance of passive house design is to reduce the energy use for heating to less than 15 kWh/(m^{2}a), which is sometimes described as a technical standard. For lowering transmissible energy losses through the transparent parts of the building envelope, the declared light transmittance (i.e., the proportion of the visible light spectrum that is transmitted through the glass) for glazing is at least 0.5. This value applies to idle conditions with perpendicular radiation and clean surfaces on both sides of the glazing. Considering these two factors, a more realistic value of light transmittance is 0.36. In order to evaluate the effect of light transmittance on the heat and daylight balance of the building, Krainer (2008) carried out a comparative analysis of 27 randomly selected buildings using the aforementioned windows.

BOX 1.6 Study evidence

"In a passive house, energy use for heating was reduced, on average, by 15% annually, while average daylight illuminance was lower by 25% on average, compared to a bioclimatic house. In the worst case scenario, the reduction in energy use for heating was 13%, and the worsening of daylight illuminance was by 60%!" (Krainer 2008, p. 402). The lack of daylight in built environments has adverse effects on health, comfort and productivity (Nicklas and Bailey 1997; Hathaway et al. 1992).

One of the implemented partial measures towards energy efficiency is often the installation of highly efficient mechanical systems, but with a lack of other holistic bioclimatic measures, which should be taken into account as priority actions. As a result, the savings are minimal.

BOX 1.7 Study evidence

The study on exergy consumption patterns for space heating in Slovenian buildings (Dovjak et al. 2010, p. 3004) showed that interventions performed on building envelope systems resulted in 6.25 times higher total building exergy saving potential than interventions in the efficiency of mechanical systems. Additionally, the combination of building system improvements and occupant's behavioural changes resulted in a reduction of 75–95% of exergy consumption of heating and cooling (Schweiker and Shukuya 2010, p. 2983). Simple actions have influence not only on significant energy savings but also on improved thermal comfort conditions (Shukuya 2009, p. 1550) and occupant's behavioural changes (Schweiker and Shukuya, 2010, p. 2976).

As the built environment is for people living there, we need to have a better understanding of the nature of occupants, i.e., occupant behaviour and it is necessary to design the built environment so as to have the occupants be healthy and comfortable enough with less exergy consumption in heating or cooling systems (Shukuya 2013, p. 108).

In HVAC systems, recuperators are commonly used to re-use waste heat from exhaust air normally expelled to the atmosphere. Such devices typically comprise a series of parallel plates of aluminium, plastic, stainless steel, or synthetic fibre, alternate pairs of which are enclosed on two sides to form twin sets of ducts at right angles to each other, and which contain the supply and extract air streams. In this manner, heat from the exhaust air stream is transferred through the separating plates, and into the supply air stream. Manufacturers claim gross efficiencies of up to 80% depending upon the specification of the unit (Milovančevič and Kosi 2016; Albers 2016). Many users report installation problems:

BOX 1.8 Opinion evidence

Some of the important disadvantages of the installed recuperator are noise and dry air. Moreover, it stopped working after 2 months of usage, because of clogged air filters.

Another example is the installation of heat pumps, which are often advertised as economical and environmentally friendly technologies. The heat pump extracts the heat from its environment and passes it on, the reverse principle to refrigerating. The heat of the groundwater, the ground or the atmosphere is absorbed by the refrigerant and used to supply heat after compression (Albers 2016). Heat pumps can be used for space heating or providing domestic hot water. Users report difficulties with installation and functioning:

BOX 1.9 Opinion evidence

A heat pump does not produce water as hot as a boiler with a maximum flow temperature of 55 °C. Low temperatures result in greater energy savings, but they presented a critical point in complete control and prevention against *Legionella* spp. So, from that perspective thermal disinfection is not possible at all. Also, heat pumps are often shut down during summer period.

In accordance with the requirements for water sanitation, the measurements for complete control and prevention against *Legionella* spp. should be performed (OJ RS, No. 19/2004; OJ RS, No. 88/2012; Joseph et al. 2005; Bartram et al. 2007; NIJZ 2017; HSE 2000). One such important measure is about water temperature; temperatures between 20 and 50 °C are favourable for the growth and reproduction of *Legionella* spp. Keeping the water temperature outside the ideal range for legionellae is an effective control measure for both hot and cold-water systems (WHO 2017).

Designers are mostly familiar with the specific requirements that are under their jurisdiction. It often happens that they do not cooperate with other experts during the planning and design process. Requirements are often unilateral, excluding or contradicting each other. As an example, we should mention the Slovenian national legislation, the rules on ventilation and air-conditioning of buildings (OJ RS, No. 42/2002, chang.) define a minimum number of air changes per hour per room (living, working) at 0.5. Fulfilment of this requirement results in decreased ventilation losses and inadequate indoor air quality.

Design should be in the direction towards healthy and comfortable indoor environments with the lowest possible energy use and not the lowest energy use based on the physiological minimum (Krainer 2008, p. 399).

Measures taken to improve building energy efficiency rarely consider their impact on indoor environmental quality. The same problem was highlighted in the study by Földváry et al. (2017), who evaluated the impact of simple energy renovation on indoor air quality, air exchange rates, and occupant satisfaction in Slovak residential buildings:

BOX 1.10 Study evidence

Földváry et al. (2017, p. 363) showed that CO_2 concentrations were significantly higher and air exchange rates were lower in renovated buildings. Formaldehyde concentrations increased after renovation and were positively correlated with CO_2 and relative air humidity. Energy renovation was associated with lower occupant satisfaction with indoor air quality.

Hribar et al. (2017) performed a case study on multi-dwelling residential building in which the effect of an increased number of air changes (from 0.7 ach to 1.0 ach) was evaluated from energy and air quality perspectives:

BOX 1.11 Study evidence

Building case with a higher number of air changes (1 ach) resulted in a minimal increase of total energy use (heating, cooling, lighting, interior heat sources) compared to the building case with the lower number of air changes (0.7 ach) (2.63% changes). Additionally, a higher number of air changes (1 ach) resulted in considerable improvement in indoor air quality parameter, CO_2 (30.0% changes) (Hribar et al. 2017, p. 29).

In Slovenia, the problem of minimization of ventilation losses by minimal permissible design ventilation rates was highlighted by Dovjak et al. (2019). Such approach is supported by national legislation that often allows the use of minimal permissible values for ventilation, while other required and recommended optimal values are not taken into consideration:

BOX 1.12 Study evidence
In the work titled "Deteriorated Indoor Environmental Quality as a Collateral Damage of Present Day Extensive Renovations" (Dovjak et al. 2019), a combination of simulations of selected parameters of indoor air quality and building energy use was performed for five sets of scenarios, where design ventilation rates varied according to national legislation. Characteristics of actual kindergarten in central Slovenia, renovated in 2016, were used for building model and performed simulations. The results showed that minimal permissible value, ACH 0.5, results in the highest concentration of CO_2 in both model playrooms that exceeded the national maximum permissible level for acceptable indoor air quality by 2.5 times and 3 times, and the recommended value for Category I by 5.6 times and 6.6 times. Formaldehyde concentrations in both model playrooms reached almost the value recommended by WHO (World Health Organization) and exceeded the level recommended by NIOSH (National Institute for Occupational Safety and Health, CDC) by 4.6 and 4.5 times. The required and recommended design ventilation rates have to be in-line with scientific findings that support higher required design ventilation rates to attain optimal indoor air quality (Dovjak et al. 2019, p. 31). Design ventilation rates have to consider the highest amount of fresh air per person (i.e. actual number of occupants) and the highest amount of fresh air per m^2 due to possible emissions. At the first stage of design, it is important to select non-toxic construction products (Dovjak et al. 2019, p. 38).

Nevertheless, the required and/or recommended thermal comfort parameters (i.e., air temperature, operative temperature, surface temperature, relative humidity) are mainly based on characteristics of an average person (i.e., a 30-year old male, weighing 70 kg, and 1.75 m tall; a 30-year old female, weighing 60 kg and 1.70 m tall) and do not satisfy individual needs, as proven with studies by Hwang et al. (2007), Mallick (1996), Nicol (2004). Moreover, in every environment, vulnerable population groups are always present. Designing indoor conditions based on averages results in uncomfortable or even unhealthy conditions for many people.

Finally, the subjects that are involved in the design process often act independently without including other professionals in different design stages. Due to the lack of knowledge on specific issues, some non-functional solutions are developed (e.g., dysfunctional layouts of health facilities, as pointed out by employees).

BOX 1.13 Opinion evidence
Due to financial cutbacks, the initial layouts for the ambulance room size were minimized, between corridors and inspection rooms curtains were installed and not doors, many rooms are without windows, there is a huge lack of privacy, manoeuvring patients is not possible, there is a lack of daylight and poor indoor air quality.

In this health institution, the layouts were designed without consideration of the actual number of users (e.g., patient, staff), specifics of working process and installed devices (e.g., number, sizes, layout). Such active spaces do not serve the purpose for which they were designed.

1.6 Most Common Problems in the Built Environment— Epidemiological Data

The WHO estimated that the environment, as a major health determinant, accounts for almost 20% of all deaths in the WHO European Region. A degraded urban environment, with air and noise pollution and lack of green spaces and mobility options, also poses health risks (WHO 2017; WHO Europe 2007). Housing-related inequalities are one of the environmental health inequality indicators set by the WHO. Inadequate housing conditions exist in all sub-regions and in all countries and are most often suffered by disadvantaged population groups. The WHO estimates for 11 housing hazards, related, for example, to noise, damp, indoor air quality, cold, and home safety, show that in the WHO European Region inadequate housing accounts for over 100,000 deaths per year.

There are 18–50% of buildings on a global scale, and 18% of buildings in Europe with excessive indoor moisture and humidity problems (Mudarri and Fisk 2007). In Europe, 15% of the general population is affected by dampness in the home in the EU15 (for the 15 Member States belonging to the EU before May 2004) versus 18% in the NMS12 countries (for the 12 Member States joining the EU after May 2004). However, within these regional averages, strong national variations are observed. The lowest prevalence is found in Finland, where only 5% of the population live in damp homes; similarly, low levels were found in Sweden and Slovakia. Slovenia has the highest prevalence at 30%, followed by Cyprus at 29%; 32.4% of people in Slovenia live in homes with leafy roofs, damp walls and floor bases, damaged window frames or floors (National Housing Program 2015–2025 2015). In some European countries, 20–30% of households have problems with damp, which increases the risk of respiratory disorders by 50%.

The inability to keep homes warm constitutes a housing issue among both the new Member State (NMS12) countries (18.4% prevalence among the general population) and—although to a lesser extent—the EU15 countries (6.9% prevalence). Globally, the proportion of the general population unable to keep their dwellings comfortably cool in summer is higher than the proportion unable to keep their homes warm in winter, showing that summer temperatures may be a rising problem. Much higher prevalence levels can be found among NMS12 countries (average 37.7%) than among the EU15 countries (average 24.2%).

The overall prevalence of complaints about noise from neighbours or from the street varies by country between 10 and 35%, with an average of 22% across the EU27 (WHO 2009). About every tenth lung cancer case results from radon in the home. Poor design or construction of homes is the cause of most home accidents. In some European countries, home accidents kill more people than road accidents do. Appropriate design can prevent both exposure and the risk to health.

Other adverse effects of the built environment on health, comfort, and wellbeing: Users are exposed to numerous adverse health effects that are directly or indirectly related to the quality of the environment. Environmental stressors (i.e., environmental factor intensities severe enough to require a compensatory response at any level of biological mechanisms, Wedemeyer and Goodyear 1984), such as chemical stressors (e.g., air quality) or physical stressors (e.g., noise, light, air temperature), can affect human bodies throughout the life cycle, including the prenatal phase. Environmental stressors can affect health on various levels including gene modification, changes in cellular activity and growth, changes in specific processes in tissue or the body. Consequently, regarding the type of the stressor, dose, duration of exposure, and vulnerability, the exposure can lead to the occurrence and development of the disease or its exacerbation. Asthma, allergies, temperature-related impacts on comfort and human performance, are disorders of circadian rhythms are examples of adverse effects caused by stressors in built environments.

Global results show that **asthma** has a higher prevalence in low-income urban communities with high levels of air pollution, poor indoor air quality, as well as in water-damaged, mouldy homes (EPA 2017b; Münzel and Daiber 2018). Research shows that asthma disproportionately impacts minority children; however, it is a common disease found in people over age 65. In the built environment, indoor air pollution and other kinds of contamination can lead to or exacerbate asthma (EPA 2017b). Design of buildings must consider these issues in order to reduce environmental stressors in built environments and help in asthma prevention (EPA 2017b; Jantunen et al. 2011).

Allergies are accepted as a significant public health problem that is frequently observed worldwide (Gül and Atli 2014). It is characterized by an abnormal immune response to environmental antigens, which are frequently encountered. The World Allergy Organization reported that 22% of the participants in global scale studies suffered from at least one allergy (Warner et al. 2006). In recent years, there has been an increase in the prevalence of allergic diseases, especially in developed countries (Hong et al. 2012). Risk factors for an allergy can be evaluated in two categories: host factors and environmental factors. Environmental factors related to the built environment that can trigger the disease are indoor and outdoor air pollution, chemicals, mould, and dust exposure, etc. Defining and avoiding the allergen in built environments is the most efficient approach for the prevention and protection against environmental allergic diseases (Gül and Atli 2014).

Environmental stressors, specifically parameters of thermal comfort, might cause **temperature-related effects**. According to Ikäheimo (2013), the effect of heat and cold exposure on the human body include unpleasant sensations (cold, pain, hot), decreased performance (physical and cognitive), symptoms, morbidity (cardiovascular and respiratory diseases), injuries (frostbite, hypothermia, hyperthermia, heat stroke), and mortality. The risks of extreme temperature conditions on health have been growing over the years, especially due to increased frequency of extreme weather events due to climate change. Populations vulnerable to heat and cold are the elderly, those with chronic diseases, children, and socially isolated persons.

The FINRISK 2007 study (Näyhä et al. 2014) examined the ambient temperatures considered to be hot and the upper limit of comfortable and the prevalence of heat-related complaints and symptoms in the Finnish population (N = 4007, 25–74 yrs.). The authors highlighted that a large percentage of the studied population suffers from heat-related complaints (signs or symptoms of heat strain, thirst, drying of mouth, impaired endurance and sleep disturbances, cardiac and respiratory symptoms). The temperature considered to be hot averaged 26 °C and the upper limit for thermal comfort was 22 °C. Both temperatures declined with age by 1–5 °C (Näyhä et al. 2014). The PHEWE-project (Michelozzi et al. 2009) evaluated the impact of high environmental temperatures on hospital admissions in 12 European cities. For a 1 °C increase in maximum apparent temperature above a threshold, respiratory admissions increased by +4.5% and +3.1% in the 75+ age group in Mediterranean and North-Continental cities, respectively. The association between temperature and cardiovascular and cerebrovascular admissions did not reach statistical significance. WHO MONICA (Barnett et al. 2007) analysed the effect of temperature on systolic blood pressure on 25 populations in 16 countries (N = 115, 434). The results proved that a 1 °C decrease in temperature increases blood pressure. Additionally, it was highlighted that indoor temperature also correlated with blood pressure. The temperature of the environment might also have a significant effect on work performance. A review of worldwide studies by Seppänen et al. (2003) found no significant relationship of temperature to productivity in the comfort zone but reported an average 2% decrease in work performance per degree Celsius temperature rise, when the temperature was above 25 °C. The bioclimatic design of built environments is a critical action in managing heat and cold.

Daylight as a positive environmental stressor regulates our circadian rhythm (i.e., a biological process that displays an endogenous, entrainable oscillation of about 24 h). Several characteristics of light interact to influence circadian functions, including quantity, spectrum, spatial distribution, timing, and duration. Current design practice often results in too low indoor daylight levels, which consequently affect our circadian systems.

In particular, the blue part of the light spectrum affects alertness both indirectly, by modifying circadian rhythms, and directly, giving rise to acute effects. A systematic review of 68 empirical studies by Souman et al. (2018) identified that increasing the intensity of polychromatic white light was found to increase subjective ratings of alertness in a majority of studies. Additionally, inadequate daylit buildings might have an impact on the sleep quality. Düzgün and Durmaz (2017) determined the effect of light therapy on sleep problems and slept quality of elderly people (N = 61, from Social Security Institution Narlıdere Municipal Nursing Home, Turkey). The authors highlighted that the exposure to direct sunlight between 8 AM and 10 AM for 5 days seems to be effective in increasing the sleep quality. Rea et al. (2002) highlighted that the design practice, as well as the industry, should begin to optimize light's quantity, spectrum, spatial distribution, timing and duration to support circadian system functions as well as visual system functions.

1.7 Main Objectives of Planning

The main objectives of healthy and sustainable building planning and well-being are:

- To understand the human-building-environment relationship with emphasis on the health of users
- To know and define basic concepts and terminology
- To understand interconnections between natural processes inside the human body and technological processes inside the built environment (anatomical, physiological, pathological bases)
- To understand why the health and productivity of users is more important the energy use in buildings
- What the consequences are if we do not follow the basic principles of the design process
- Legal and moral responsibility
- To know how to collaborate with different profiles/sectors in the process of building design
- Support the suggestions with scientifically supported facts and evidence-based practices
- To know how to choose the right research studies and be critical to existing studies and claims in the media.

The most important goal is to design a healthy, comfortable building for living and working environments with minimal energy use and without negative environmental impacts. Furthermore, it is essential to create optimal conditions for users that promote health, comfort and greater productivity, and at the same time energy efficiency with minimal environmental impact. It is a highly complex and demanding process that requires experts with technical skills and knowledge in physiology, anatomy, health, etc. Consequently, a multidisciplinary cooperation approach between disciplines and professions as well as constructive communication is needed.

> **Citizens and politicians, bankers and lawyers, engineers and planners, designers and scientists are all indispensable and influential parts in the design, planning and management of a quality environment for all** (Bartuska 2007, p. 5)

> **One of the most important stakeholders, actively involved in participatory design of built environment, are users that live and work there** (Mahabadi et al. 2014).

References

Abbacan-Tuguic, L. (2016). Vernacular architecture: Upholding tradition through mathematical expression of artistry in the construction of Kalinga houses. *International Journal of Advanced Research in Management and Social Sciences, 5*(6), 753–773.

Albers, K. J. (2016). Taschenbuch für Heizung + Klimatechnik 2017/2018. Verlag, Vulkan-Verlag.

ANSI/ASHRAE/ASHE Standard 170-2008. (2012). Ventilation of health care facilities. Retrieved October 10, 2018 from https://www.ashrae.org/.../docLib/.../170_2008_addendum_r_Final.pdf.

ANSI/ASHRAE Standard 55. (2013). Thermal environmental conditions for human occupancy. American Society of Heating, Refrigerating and Air-Conditioning Engineers Inc., Atlanta, GA.

ASHRAE Handbook. (2007). HVAC applications: Health care facilities. American Society of Heating, Refrigerating and Air–Conditioning Engineers Inc., Atlanta, GA (p. 1039).

Barnett, A. G., Sans, S., Salomaa, V., Kuulasmaa, K., Dobson, A. J. (2007). WHO MONICA Project. The effect of temperature on systolic blood pressure. *Blood Pressure Monitoring, 12*(3), 195–203. http://dx.doi.org/10.1097/MBP.0b013e3280b083f4.

Bartram, J., Chartier, Y., Lee, J. V., Pond, K., & Surman-Lee, S. (2007). *Legionella and the prevention of legionellosis.* WHO.

Bartuska, T. J. (2007). Introduction: Definition, design, and development of the built environment. In McClure, W. R. & Bartuska, T. J. (Eds.), *The built environment: A collaborative inquiry into design and planning* (pp. 3–14). Wiley, New Jersey.

Blecich, P., Franković, M., & Kristl, Ž. (2016). Energy retrofit of the Krsan Castle: From sustainable to responsible design: A case study. *Energy and Buildings, 122,* 23–33. https://doi.org/10.1016/j.enbuild.2016.04.011.

Boundless. (2017). Urban planning in the Greek High Classical Period. Boundless Art History Boundless. Retrieved October 10, 2018 from https://www.boundless.com/art-history/textbooks/boundless-art-history-textbook/ancient-greece-6/the-high-classical-period-66/urban-planning-in-the-greek-high-classical-period-344-10749.

BPIE. (2015). Buildings performance institute Europe. In Kunkel, S., Kontonasiou, E., Arcipowska, A., Mariottini, F., & Atanasiu, B. (Eds.), *Analysis of residential building regulations in eight EU member states.* Retrieved December 3, 2018 from http://bpie.eu/wp-content/uploads/2015/10/BPIE__IndoorAirQuality2015.pdf.

Brown, J. P., & Rose, W. B. (1996). Humidity and moisture in historic buildings: The origins of building and object conservation. *APT Bulletin, 27*(3), 12–24. Retrieved October 10, 2018 from http://cool.conservationus.org/byauth/brownjp/humidity1997.html.

BS 5454. (2000). Recommendations for storage and exhibition of archival documents.

Carlson, C., Aytur, S., Gardner, K., & Rogers, S. (2012). Complexity in built environment, health, and destination walking: A neighborhood-scale analysis. *Journal of Urban Health, 89,* 270–284. https://doi.org/10.1007/s11524-011-9652-8.

CIC. (2017). Construction industry council 2017. Retrieved October 10, 2018 from http://cic.org.uk/services/all-party-parliamentary-group.php.

Climate policy info hub. (2017). Energy efficiency policy instruments in the European union. Retrieved March 13, 2017 from http://climatepolicyinfohub.eu/energy-efficiency-policy-instruments-european-union#footnote2_f4q7isw.

Constitution RS (Ustava Republike Slovenije). Retrieved October 10, 2018 from http://www.usrs.si/media/ustava.republike.slovenije.pdf.

Council Directive 92/75/EEC of 22 September 1992 on the indication by labelling and standard product information of the consumption of energy and other resources by household appliances.

CPR 305/2011 (Construction Products Regulation, No. 305/2011)/EU Regulation (EU) No 305/2011 of the European Parliament and of the Council of 9 March 2011 laying down harmonised conditions for the marketing of construction products an repealing Council Directive 89/106/EEC. Retrieved October 10, 2018 from http://eurlex.europa.eu/legalcontent/SL/TXT/?uri=CELEX%3A32011R0305.

CR 1752. (1998). *Ventilation for buildings: Design criteria for the indoor environment.* CEN, Brussels.

Crowe, N. (1997). *Nature and the idea of a man-made world: An investigation into the evolutionary roots of form and order in the built environment.* Cambridge: MIT Press.

CSIP. (2014). Conservation and collections care. CSIP environmental standards. Relative humidity and temperature parameters. Retrieved October 10, 2018 from http://conservation.myspecies.info/node/42.

Directive 89/391/EEC - OSH "Framework Directive" Council Directive 89/391/EEC of 12 June 1989 on the introduction of measures to encourage improvements in the safety and health of workers at work.

Directive 2009/28/EC of the European parliament and of the Council of 23 April 2009 on the promotion of the use of energy from renewable sources and amending and subsequently repealing Directives 2001/77/EC and 2003/30/EC.

Directive 2009/125/EC Establishing a framework for the setting of Eco-design requirements for energy-related products (recast). Official Journal of the European Union L 285/10.

Directive (EU) 2018/844 of the European Parliament and of the Council of 30 May 2018 amending Directive 2010/31/EU on the energy performance of buildings and Directive 2012/27/EU on energy efficiency.

Directive 2012/27/EU of the European Parliament and of the Council of 25 October 2012 on energy efficiency amending Directives 2009/125/EC and 2010/30/EU and repealing Directives 2004/8/EC and 2006/32/EC.

Dovjak, M., Shukuya, M., Olesen, B. W., & Krainer, A. (2010). Analysis on exergy consumption patterns for space heating in Slovenian buildings. *Energy Policy, 38*(6), 2998–3007. https://doi.org/10.1016/j.enpol.2010.01.039.

Dovjak, M. (2012). Individualization of personal space in hospital environment: Doctoral dissertation. University of Nova Gorica, Nova Gorica (p. 184). Retrieved October 10, 2018 from http://www.ung.si/ ~ library/doktorati/okolje/26Dovjak.pdf.

Dovjak, M., Kukec, A., Kristl, Ž., Košir, M., Bilban, M., Shukuya, M., et al. (2013). Integral control of health hazards in hospital environment. *Indoor and Built Environment, 22*(5), 776–795. https://doi.org/10.1177/1420326X12459867.

Dovjak, M., Krainer, A., & Shukuya, M. (2014). Individualisation of personal space in hospital environment. *International Journal of Exergy, 14*(2), 125–155. https://doi.org/10.1504/IJEX.2014.060279.

Dovjak, M., Shukuya, M., & Krainer, A. (2018). User-centred healing-oriented conditions in the design of hospital environments. *International Journal of Environmental Research and Public Health, 15*(10), 2140:1-28. http://dx.doi.org/10.3390/ijerph15102140.

Dovjak, M., Slobodnik, J., & Krainer, A. (2019). Deteriorated indoor environmental quality as a collateral damage of present day extensive renovations. *Strojniški vestnik - Journal of Mechanical Engineering, 65*(1), 31–40. https://doi.org/10.5545/sv-jme.2018.5384.

Düzgün, G., & Durmaz, A. A. (2017). Effect of natural sunlight on sleep problems and sleep quality of the elderly staying in the nursing home. *Holistic Nursing Practice, 31*(5), 295–302.

EC. (2016). European commission—fact sheet. Putting energy efficiency first: Consuming better, getting cleaner. Brussels, 30 November 2016. Retrieved March 13, 2018 from https://ec.europa.eu/energy/en/topics/energy-efficiencyMEMO-16-3986_EN.pdf.

EC. (2017). European commission energy. Buildings. Retrieved November 3, 2018 from https://ec.europa.eu/energy/en/topics/energy-efficiency/buildings.

EC 2020 – 2020 climate & energy package. Retrieved March 13, 2018 from https://ec.europa.eu/clima/policies/strategies/2020_en.

EC 2030 – 2030. Energy strategy. Retrieved October 10, 2018 from https://ec.europa.eu/energy/en/topics/energy-strategy-and-energy-union/2030-energy-strategy.

ECF. (2010). Roadmap 2050. European climate foundation. Retrieved March 13, 2018 from www.roadmap2050.euexplained/index.php/Greenhouse_gas_emissions_by_industries_and_households.

EN 15251:2007 Indoor environmental input parameters for design and assessment of energy performance of buildings addressing indoor air quality, thermal environment, lighting and acoustics.

EPA. (2017a). Energy and the environment. National action plan for energy efficiency. Retrieved October 10, 2018 from https://www.epa.gov/energy/national-action-plan-energy-efficiency.

EPA. (2017b). Asthma research. Retrieved July 9, 2018 from https://www.epa.gov/healthresearch/asthma-research.

EPBD proposal. (2016). Proposal for a directive of the european parliament and of the council amending Directive 2010/31/EU on the energy performance of buildings. Retrieved March 13, 2018 from https://ec.europa.eu/energy/sites/ener/files/documents/1_en_act_part1_v10.pdf.

EPBD-r 2010/31/EU. Directive 2010/31/EU of the European Parliament and of the Council of 19 May 2010 on the Energy Performance of Buildings (recast).

European Parliament. (2016). Directorate general for internal policies policy department A: Economic and scientific policy. In Artola, I., Rademaekers, K., Williams, R., & Yearwood, J. (Eds.), *Boosting building renovation: What potential and value for Europe?* Retrieved March 13, 2018 from http://www.europarl.europa.eu/RegData/etudes/STUD/2016/587326/IPOL_STU(2016)587326_EN.pdf.

European Social Charter (OJ RS, No. 24/1999 with chang.).

European Convention on Human Rights (ECHR).

Földváry, V., Bekö, G., Langer, S., Arrhenius, K., & Petráš, D. (2017). Effect of energy renovation on indoor air quality in multifamily residential buildings in Slovakia. *Building and Environment, 122*, 363–372. https://doi.org/10.1016/j.buildenv.2017.06.009.

Glaeser, E. (2011). *Triumph of the city: How our best invention makes us richer, smarter, greener, healthier, and happier* (p. 19). New York: Penguin Press.

Glanz, K., Handy, S. L., Henderson, K. E., Slater, S. J., Davis, E. L., & Powell, L. M. (2016). Built environment assessment: Multidisciplinary perspectives. *SSM-Population Health, 2*, 24–31.

Goldstein, B. (2002). The environment and health: A conversation with CDC chief Jeffrey Koplan; tracing the intersections between behaviour and environment fascinates this top health officer. *Health Affair, 21*, 179–184.

Gostin, L. O. (2000). Public health law: Power, duty, restraint. Berkeley, Calif: University of California Press and Milbank Memorial Fund.

Gül, H., & Atli, Z. C. (2014). Occupational and environmental risk factors for allergic and hypersensitivity reactions. Retrieved July 9, 2018 from https://pdfs.semanticscholar.org/9467/d058d85098e89ad181d0e1cff609507cedac.pdf?_ga=2.132812173.2061439577.1531468766-1738562617.1531468766.

Hathaway, W. E., Hargreaves, J. A., Thomson, G. W., & Novintsky, D. (1992). A summary of light related studies. A study into the effects of light on children of elementary school age-a case of daylight robbery. Retrieved September 17, 2018 from http://www.naturallighting.com/cart/store.php?sc_page=62.

Hong, S., Son, D. K., Lim, W. R., Kim, S. H., Kim, H., Yum, H. Y., et al. (2012). The prevalence of atopic dermatitis, asthma, and allergic rhinitis and the comorbidity of allergic diseases in children. *Environ Health Toxicol, 27,* e2012006. https://doi.org/10.5620/eht.2012.27.e2012006.

Hribar, B., Poglajen, S., Nizandžić, A., & Petrič, A. (2017). Energy efficiency and indoor environmental quality: Case study. Faculty of Civil and Geodetic Engineering, University of Ljubljana, Ljubljana.

HSE. (2000). Legionnaires' disease: The control of legionella bacteria in water systems. HSE Approved code of practice & guidance.

Hudobivnik, B., Pajek, L., Kunič, R., & Košir, M. (2016). FEM thermal performance analysis of multi-layer external walls during typical summer conditions considering high intensity passive cooling. *Applied Energy, 178,* 363–375. https://doi.org/10.1016/j.apenergy.2016.06.036.

Hwang, R. L., Lin, T. P., Cheng, M. J., & Chien, J. H. (2007). Patient thermal comfort requirement for hospital environments in Taiwan. *Building and Environment, 42*(8), 2980–2987. https://doi.org/10.1016/j.buildenv.2006.07.035.

IPPC. (2018). Projections of future changes in climate. Retrieved July 9, 2018 from https://www.ipcc.ch/publications_and_data/ar4/wg1/en/spmsspm-projections-of.html.

ISO 7730. (2005). Ergonomics of the thermal environment–Analytical determination and interpretation of thermal comfort using calculation of the PMV and PPD indices and local thermal comfort criteria.

ISO/TC 205/WG 002 (1998). Building environmental design.

Ikäheimo, T. M. (2013). The effects of temperature on human health. Retrieved July 9, 2018 from http://www.oulu.fi/sites/default/files/content/Ikaheimo_TM_Temperature_and_human_health_28102014.pdf.

Jantunen, M., Oliveira Fernandes, E., Carrer, P., & Kephalopoulos, S. (2011). Promoting actions for healthy indoor air (IAIAQ) European Commission Directorate General for Health and Consumers. Luxembourg. Retrieved October 10, 2018 from https://ec.europa.eu/health//sites/health/files/healthy_environments/docs/env_iaiaq.pdf.

Joseph, C., Lee, J., van Wijngaarden, J., Drasar, V., & Castellani-Pastoris, M. (2005). European Guidelines for the control and prevention of travel associated legionnaires' disease. The European surveillance scheme for travel associated legionnaires disease and the European working group for legionella infections, 2005.

Kent, J. L., & Thompson, S. (2014). The three domains of urban planning for health and well-being. *Journal of Planning Literature, 29*(3), 239–256.

Kunič, R. (2017). Carbon footprint of thermal insulation materials in building envelopes. *Energy Efficiency, 10,* 1511–1528. https://doi.org/10.1007/s12053-017-9536-1.

Kunič, R. (2016). Forest-based bioproducts used for construction and its impact on the environmental performance of a building in the whole life cycle. In Kutnar, A., & Muthu, S. S. (Eds.), *Environmental impacts of traditional and innovative forest-based bioproducts. Environmental footprints and Eco-design of products and processes* (pp. 173–204). Singapore: Springer.

Kuzman Kitek, M., & Kutnar, A. (2014). *Contemporary Slovenian timber architecture for sustainability.* Cham: Springer.

Krainer, A. (1993a). Vernacular buildings in Slovenia: Genesis of bioclimatic growth of vernacular buildings in Slovenia, European Commission. TEMPUS Programme (p. 102).

Krainer, A. (1993b). *Toward smart buildings, (Building science and environment-conscious design, Module 1: Design principles, 7).* European Commission, London.

Krainer, A. (2008). Passivhaus contra design = Dedicated to em. Univ.-Prof. Dr. Ing. habil. Dr.h.c. mult. Karl Gertis on the occasion of his 70th birthday. *Bauphysik, 30*(6), 393–404. http://dx. doi.org/10.1002/bapi.200810051.

Mallick, F. H. (1996). Thermal comfort and building design in the tropical climates. *Energy and Buildings, 23*(3), 161–167. https://doi.org/10.1016/0378-7788(95)00940-X.

Mahabadi, S. M., Zabihi, H., & Majedi, H. (2014). Participatory design; a new approach to regenerate the public space. *International Journal of Architecture and Urban Development, 4* (4), 15–22.

Maynard, D. N., & Hochmuth, G. J. (2007). *Knott's handbook for vegetable growers* (5th ed.). New Jersey: Wiley.

McClure, W. R., & Bartuska, T. J. (2007). *The built environment: A collaborative inquiry into design and planning.* New Jersey: Wiley.

Melillo, J. M., Richmond, T., & Yohe, G.W. (2014). Climate change impacts in the United States: The third national climate assessment. U.S. Global Change Research Program, Washington, DC.

Michelozzi, P., Accetta, G., De Sario, M., D'Ippoliti, D., Marino, C., Baccini, M., et al., PHEWE Collaborative Group. (2009). High temperature and hospitalizations for cardiovascular and respiratory causes in 12 European cities. *American Journal of Respiratory and Critical Care Medicine, 179*(5), 383–389. http://dx.doi.org/10.1164/rccm.200802-217OC.

Milovančevič, U., & Kosi, F. (2016). Performance analysis of system heat pump—Heat recuperator used for air treatment in process industry. *Thermal Science, 20*(4), 1345–1354.

Mokdad, A. H., Ford, E. S., Bowman, B. A., Dietz, W. H., Vinicor, F., Bales, V. S., et al. (2003). Prevalence of obesity, diabetes, and obesity-related health risk factors, 2001. *JAMA, 289*(1), 76–79.

Mudarri, D., & Fisk, W. J. (2007). Public health and economic impact of dampness and mold. *Indoor Air, 17*(3), 226–235. https://doi.org/10.1111/j.1600-0668.2007.00474.x.

Münzel, T., & Daiber, A. (2018). Environmental stressors and their impact on health and disease with focus on oxidative stress. *Antioxidants & Redox Signaling, 28*(9), 735–740.

National Housing Program 2015–2025 (2015). RS.

National Institute of Building Sciences. (2017). An authoritative source of innovative solutions for the built environment, Washington, DC, vol. 202, 289–7800. Retrieved October 10, 2018 from https://www.wbdg.org/building-types.

Natural Building Blog. (2013). Thriving Sustainably with Earthbag Building and Other Practical Solutions Natural Building, Book III, Chapter VIII, of Xenophon's Memorabilia of Socrates, written a few decades after Aeschylus. Retrieved October 10, 2018 from http://www. naturalbuildingblog.com/sun-tempered-architecture-socrates-house/.

Näyhä, S., Rintamäki, H., Donaldson, G., Hassi, J., Jousilahti, P., Laatikainen, T., et al. (2014). Heat-related thermal sensation, comfort and symptoms in a northern population: The national FINRISK 2007 study. *The European Journal of Public Health, 24*(4), 620–626.

Nicklas, M. H., & Bailey, G. B. (1997). Analysis of the performance of students in daylit schools. In *Proceedings of the 1997 Annual Conference, ASES* (pp. 1–5). Colorado: American Solar Energy Society.

Nicol, F. (2004). Adaptive thermal comfort standards in the hot-humid tropics. *Energy and Buildings, 36,* 628–637. https://doi.org/10.1016/j.enbuild.2004.01.016.

NIJZ. (2017). National institute of public health. *Legionella* spp. water management. Retrieved October 10, 2018 from http://www.nijz.si/sl/preprecevanje-razmnozevanja-legionel-v-hisnem-vodovodnem-omrezju.

OJ RS, No. 89/1999, chang.: Rules on requirements for ensuring safety and health of workers at workplaces.

OJ RS, No. 73/2000, chang.: Rules on standards and minimal technical conditions for kindergarten premises and equipment.

OJ RS, No. 90/2001: Order on the living conditions and supply of wildlife species in captivity.

OJ RS, No. 42/2002, chang.: Rules on the ventilation and air-conditioning of buildings.

OJ RS, No. 19/2004, chang.: Rules on drinking water.

OJ RS, No. 88/2012: Decree on drinking water supply.

OJ RS, No. 61/2017, chang.: Building Act.

OJ RS, No. 37/2018: Decree on Classification of Construction.

Pajek, L., Hudobivnik, B., Kunič, R., & Košir, M. (2017). Improving thermal response of lightweight timber building envelopes during cooling season in three European locations. *Journal of Cleaner Production, 156,* 939–952. https://doi.org/10.1016/j.jclepro.2017.04.098.

Perdue, C. W., Stone, L. A., & Gostin, L. O., JD, LLD (Hon). (2003). The built environment and its relationship to the public's health: The legal framework. *American Journal of Public Health, 93*(9), 1390–1394.

Rea, M. S., Figueiro, M. G., & Bullough, J. D. (2002). Circadian photobiology: An emerging framework for lighting practice and research. *Lighting Research and Technology, 34,* 177–187. https://doi.org/10.1191/1365782802lt057oa.

Reinhard, S. C., Given, B., Petlick, N. H., & Bemis, A. (2008). Chapter 14. Supporting family caregivers in providing care. In Hughes, R. G. (Eds.), *Patient safety and quality: An evidence-based handbook for nurses.* Agency for Healthcare Research and Quality, U.S. Department of Health and Human Services, US.

Renalds, A., Smith, T., & Hale, P. (2010). A systematic review of built environment and health. *Family and Community Health, 33,* 68–78. https://doi.org/10.1097/FCH.0b013e3181c4e2e5.

Roadmap 2050 Energy Roadmap 2050, Impact assessment and scenario analysis. Commission staff working paper, Impact assessment, Accompanying the document, Communication from the commission to the council, the European Parliament, the European economic and social committee and the committee of the regions, energy roadmap 2050. Brussel, 2011. Retrieved October 10, 2018 from http://ec.europa.eu/smart-regulation/impact/ia_carried_out/docs/ia_2014/swd_2014_0015_en.pdf.

Roof, K., & Oleru, N. (2008). Public health: Seattle and King County's push for the built environment. *Journal of Environmental Health, 71,* 24–27.

Rosen, G. (1993). *A history of public health* (pp. 177–178, 212–213, 314–316). Baltimore: Johns Hopkins University, Johns Hopkins University Press.

Scott, W. H. (1996). *On the cordillera: A look at the peoples and cultures of the mountain province.* Manila: MCS Enterprises Inc.

Schickhofer, G., & Hasewend, B. (2000). Solid timber construction a construction system for residential houses, office and industrial buildings. In *Preliminary proceedings, timber frame building systems, seismic behaviour of timber buildings, timber construction in the new millennium* (p. 9), Graz. Retrieved January 2, 2019 from https://www.holzbauforschung.at/fileadmin/user_upload_hbf/News/2011/2000_Venedig_COST_E5.pdf.

Schweiker, M., & Shukuya, M. (2010). Comparative effects of building envelope improvements and occupant behavioural changes on the exergy consumption for heating and cooling. *Energy Policy, 38*(6), 2976–2986. https://doi.org/10.1016/j.enpol.2010.01.035.

Seppänen, O., Fisk, W. J., & Faulkner, D. (2003). Cost benefit analysis of the night-time ventilative cooling in office buildings. In *Conference: Healthy buildings 2003 conference,* Singapore (SG), 12/07/2003–12/11/2003.

Shukuya, M. (2009). Exergy concept and its application to the built environment. *Building and Environment, 44*(7), 1545–1550. https://doi.org/10.1016/j.buildenv.2008.06.019.

Shukuya, M. (2013). *Exergy. Theory and applications in the built environment.* Heidelberg: Springer.

Shukuya, M. (2019). *Bio-climatology for built environment* (1st ed.). Boca Raton, Florida: CRC Press, Taylor & Francis Group.

Souman, J. L., Tinga, A. M., te Pas, S. F., van Ee, R., & Vlaskamp, B. N. S. (2018). Acute alerting effects of light: A systematic literature review. *Behavioural Brain Research, 337,* 228–239. https://doi.org/10.1016/j.bbr.2017.09.016.

Stritih, U., & Koželj, R. (2017). Materials and numerical analysis of thermochemical seasonal solar energy storage for building thermal comfort applications: A review. *Research Journal of Environmental Sciences, 11*(4), 177–191. https://doi.org/10.3923/rjes.2017.177.191.

Trček Pečjak, T., & Ivanišin, M. (2017). Conservation and exhibition of paintings, Skupnost muzejev Slovenije, Ljubljana. Retrieved November 2, 2018 from http://www.sms-muzeji.si/udatoteke/publikacija/netpdf/8-4-2.pdf.

TSG-12640-001: 2008. Spatial technical guideline. TSG-12640-001: 2008. Health-care facilities. Ministry of Health, Republic of Slovenia.

USGCRP. (2016). The Impacts of climate change on human health in the United States: A scientific assessment. In Crimmins, A., Balbus, J., Gamble, J. L., Beard, C. B., Bell, J. E., Dodgen, D., et al. (Eds.), U.S. Global Change Research Program, Washington, DC.

Vitruvius Pollio, M., & Morgan, M. H. (1960). *Vitruvius: The ten books on architecture*. New York: Dover Publications.

Warner, J. O., Kaliner, M. A., Crisci, C. D., Del Giacco, S., Frew, A. J., Liu, G. H., et al., World Allergy Organization Specialty and Training Council. (2006). Allergy practice worldwide: A report by the world allergy organization specialty and training council. *International Archives of Allergy And Immunology, 139*(2), 166–174. http://dx.doi.org/10.1159/000090502.

WHO Europe. (2007). Housing and health regulations in Europe, summary document. Supported by the convention between The French Ministry of Health and World Health Organization, Regional Office for Europe with the support of the Municipality of Forlì, Italy and the Region Emilia-Romagna, Italy. Retrieved October 10, 2018 from http://www.euro.who.int/__data/assets/pdf_file/0019/121834/E89278sum.pdf.

WHO. (2009). Night noise guidelines for Europe. Retrieved October 10, 2018 from http://www.euro.who.int/__data/assets/pdf_file/0017/43316/E92845.pdf.

WHO. (2017). WHOQOL: Measuring quality of life. Retrieved October 10, 2018 from http://www.who.int/healthinfo/survey/whoqol-qualityoflife/en/.

Wedemeyer, G. A., & Goodyear, C. P. (1984). Disease caused by environmental stressors IV. In *Diseases of marine animals. Volume IV, Part 1: Introduction, pisces.* Wiley and the Biologische Anstalt Helgoland.

Working Environment (Air Pollution, Noise and Vibration) Convention, 1977 (No. 148).

Chapter 2
Health Outcomes Related to Built Environments

Abstract This chapter is dedicated to understanding the conceptual differences between healthy and unhealthy built environments (Sect. 2.1) as well as comfortable and uncomfortable conditions (Sect. 2.2) by using standardized professional terminology. In Sect. 2.3, the role of wellbeing in the sustainable building concepts is discussed and further addressed in the context of eco-friendly, green, and low-carbon buildings. The largest part of this chapter is devoted to various health effects related to exposure to health risk factors in the built environment (Sect. 2.4). In Sect. 2.5, health outcomes shown by reviewed epidemiological studies in Europe and worldwide are detailed. The chapter concludes with a determination of priority environments in public and residential buildings as well as vulnerable population groups (Sect. 2.6).

2.1 Healthy Versus Unhealthy Buildings

Health is a state of complete physical, mental and social well-being and not merely the absence of disease or infirmity (WHO 1946).

The term **health** was defined by the World Health Organization (WHO) in 1946 and entered into force on 7 April 1948. The definition has not been amended since 1948 (WHO 1946).

The definition of health has evolved. In 1948, in a radical departure from previous definitions, WHO proposed a definition that aimed higher: linking health to well-being, in terms of "physical, mental, and social well-being, and not merely the absence of disease and infirmity" (WHO 2005). Moreover, in 1986, WHO (1986) adopted a broad definition of health: "Health is a state of well-being and the capability to function in the face of changing circumstances." Currently, multiple definitions of health exist, from medical, sociological, psychological to physical definitions.

M. Dovjak and A. Kukec, *Creating Healthy and Sustainable Buildings*, https://doi.org/10.1007/978-3-030-19412-3_2

The health statuses of individuals and communities are influenced by many factors known as "health determinants". A model of wider health determinants was developed by Dahlgren and Whitehead (1991) and adapted by Barton and Grant (2006) to focus on neighbourhoods and planning. It emphasises the role of place and the built environment in contributing to health and well-being.

> According to the WHO, the main health determinants include the social and economic environment, the physical environment, and the person's individual characteristics and behaviours (WHO 2017a, p 1).

Between levels of health determinants, a continuous interaction exists (Fig. 2.1). In this respect, dynamic relationships among major influences on health and well-being were emphasized in a model created by Evans and Stoddart (1990): social environment, physical environment, genetic endowment, individual response (behaviour and biology), health care, disease, health and function, well-being, and prosperity.

According to the model of Barton and Grant (2006), the natural and built environments are critical health determinants, both of which can influence a population's health.

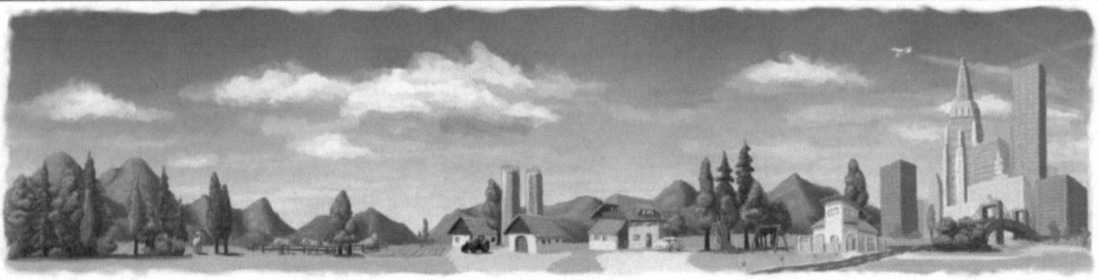

Natural environment	Individuals	Community	Built environment
• Air, water, land, soil, food • Natural habitats • Biodiversity • Global ecosystem, etc.	• Age, sex, hereditary factors • Lifestyle, diet, physical activity • Income • Culture • Activities • Work-life balance, etc.	• Social capital • Networks • Local and macro-economy, politics • Global forces • Health care service, social service, etc.	• Rural, suburban, urban • Landscape, cities, regions, Earth • Streets, routes • Products, materials • Buildings, interior, structures: active spaces, functional zones • Places • Transportation, etc.

Fig. 2.1 Conception of the health determinants and total built environment

> *A Dictionary of Epidemiology* defined the term "environment" as "all that which is external to the individual human host and it can be divided into physical, biological, social, cultural, etc." (Last 2011).

The **environment**, environmental factors (or influences) and their interactions have an essential role in creating disability, as well as the relevance of associated health conditions and their effects. Therefore, the built environment and other external factors have also been added to the **International Classification of Functioning, Disability and Health** (WHO 2001) as important determinants of health and disability.

Before we define a healthy building, environmental health should be mentioned, because it is the main element that contributes to it.

> WHO (1989) defines **environmental health** as "those aspects of human health and disease that are determined by factors in the environment".
>
> The concept of the **healthy building** was introduced by Ho et al. (2004) and defined as a "built environment that encourages positive well-being of human beings".

Environmental health includes both the direct pathological effects of chemicals, radiation, and some biological agents, and the effects (often indirect) on health and wellbeing of the broad physical, psychological, social and aesthetic environment, which includes housing, urban development, land use, and transport (Novick 1999). Environmental health also refers to the theory and practice of assessing and controlling factors in the environment that can potentially affect health. In this respect, it presents a branch of **environmental public health** that is concerned with all aspects of the natural and built environment that may affect human health. Towards the efficient control of factors that can potentially affect health, the requirements that we have to fulfil to create healthy environment must be defined. In the comprehensive work on Environmental health by Yassi et al. (2001), five basic requirements for a healthy environment were listed:

1. Clean **air**
2. Safe and sufficient **water**
3. Safe and nutritious **food**
4. Safe and peaceful **settlements**
5. A stable global **ecosystem suitable** for human habitation.

As was presented in Chap. 1 in detail, buildings are a crucial component of the total built environment as well as a health determinant. Generally, the term "healthy building" is widespread in many national and international strategies, programmes, and actions and is used as an approach in many epidemiologic or building engineering studies and projects. Ho et al. (2004) pointed out some characteristics that a healthy building should have:

- A healthy building should not be too **densely populated**
- Its window design and layout should facilitate **natural ventilation** and **diffusion of daylight**
- It should be isolated from **noise** and **air pollution** sources
- Its **water supply** and **waste systems** should be appropriately installed, maintained, and managed
- Its **environmental conditions** should be clean and hygienic.

> On the Healthy Buildings website, a **healthy building** is described as "an efficient building that allows the people within the building to operate at their highest functionality. A building is a machine that works on behalf of us humans. The goal of the building is to enable the humans working within the structure to operate at their peak efficiency. If the building enables the people within to work in a productive, happy environment, then it creates a more efficient and profitable asset for the building owner" (Turner 2016).

Numerous researchers have attempted to define the main elements and factors of healthy buildings. For example, the multifactorial elements that contribute to the healthy building by Loftness et al. (2007) were:

- Healthy, sustainable **air**
- Healthy, sustainable **thermal control**
- Healthy, sustainable **light**
- **Workplace** ergonomics and **environmental quality**
- Access to the **natural environment**
- **Land use** and **transportation**.

In a comprehensive literature review by Mao et al. (2017), the meaning of "healthy building" was defined, and 30 impact factors in the life cycle of healthy buildings were identified using bibliometric analysis and expert interviews. Additionally, on a case study of Tehran, policies and strategies for the architectural design of healthy buildings were determined: **quality of life, productivity, equity and social inclusion, environmental sustainability, and infrastructure** (Mohtashami et al. 2016). A special issue on "Sustainable and healthy buildings" was published in the journal *Energy and Buildings* (Kim 2012), in which a strategic basis for understanding how sustainable, healthy buildings can be designed, constructed, and maintained was provided.

The relationship between the health of an inhabitant and the building's state was studied in one of the largest Pan-European surveys, called Velux 2017. The survey included feedback from 14,000 respondents in 14 EU countries. For the purpose of the survey, nine indicators for healthy homes were defined, which cover:

- **Indoor air quality**
- **Daylight**
- **Sleep quality**
- **Energy costs**
- Environmental impact from **building materials**.

One of the main findings of the survey was "a healthy home is of primary importance for healthy living for Europeans" (Velux 2017, p 13).

In contrast to the terms "health" or "healthy environment", there is no standardized professional definition of a healthy building. **If we summarized the officially accepted definitions of health (WHO 1946; WHO 1989) and healthy environment (WHO 2017a), a healthy building may be better defined as**:

A healthy building is a component within a healthy built environment and is the living or working environment where all health risk factors are fully prevented, and optimal conditions for the health and wellbeing of individual users are attained. Optimal conditions include stimulating and healing-oriented conditions, which result in the fulfilment of specific needs for individual users and vulnerable ones.

An unhealthy building is a living or working environment where users are exposed to health risk factors and their parameters, without the attainment of optimal conditions for individuals, especially vulnerable ones.

At this point, the most important question is: **"Who is responsible for the design of healthy buildings within healthy built environments and, consequently, the prevention of health risk factors?"**

The Velux study determined that 42% of Europeans assign owners the highest level of responsibility (Velux 2017). Experts often have the same opinion as the general public does, despite the fact that the responsibility is shared among all involved subjects throughout the entire life cycle of the buildings, according to the CPR 305/2011. Individuals are unlikely to be able to directly control many of the health determinants in built environments. Improving health is a shared responsibility of **healthcare providers, public health experts**, and a variety of **other actors in the community** who can contribute to the well-being of individuals and populations (Institute of Medicine 1997). In this context, designers have to collaborate with experts and building users in order to provide optimal conditions for users that promote health. **Therefore, shifting the responsibility to the occupants shall not be allowed at any stage of the design of built environments.**

2.2 Comfortable Versus Uncomfortable Conditions

> Health is only possible where resources are available to **meet human needs**
> and where the living and working environment is protected from life
> threatening and health threatening pollutants, pathogens and physical hazards
> (WHO 1992).

Satisfaction of fundamental human needs (Maslow 1943) by reaching the optimal
stimulating, healthy, and comfortable conditions for each individual user (WHO
1946) is the main goal of the design of built environments.

2.2.1 Satisfaction of Human Needs in the Built Environment and the Process of Homeostasis

Every human being is daily subject to a large number of needs that arise as a result
either of some imbalances inside the body or outside factors. According to
Maslow's (1943) theory, human needs are positioned in the shape of a pyramid.
The largest and most fundamental **physiological needs** (i.e., breathing, food, water,
sleep, homeostasis, avoiding pain, sexuality, etc.) are positioned at the bottom level,
and the psychological needs (i.e., safety, love, belonging, esteem, self-actualization)
are positioned at higher levels. Maslow's theory suggests that the most basic level
of needs must be met before an individual will strongly desire (or focus motivation
upon) the secondary or higher level needs (Maslow 1943). The absence of the
fulfilment of basic needs is much more difficult to tolerate than any dissatisfaction
regarding higher needs.

Environmental parameters of thermal comfort are one of the basic physiological
needs (Maslow 1943). The physiological needs can be fulfilled with the mechanism
of homeostasis or progressively (Musek and Pečjak 2001). This is a condition for
the state of homeostasis of the human body, which enables dynamic equilibrium
within the body and its surroundings. For example, the cell membrane maintains
homeostasis through the processes of diffusion, osmosis and filtration, which are
passive forms of transport. The total daily diffusional turnover of water across all
the capillaries in the body is approx. 80.000 litres per day (Brandis 2013).

Homeostasis is maintained by regulatory mechanisms that operate through
negative feedback mechanisms (Bresjanac and Rupnik 1999; Cannon 1926).
Thermoregulation is part of the homeostatic mechanism that maintains the body's
null energy and mass balance (Bresjanac and Rupnik 1999; Cannon 1926). All
homeostatic control mechanisms have three essential components: detector, integrator, and effector. The detector monitors and responds to stimuli in the environment (i.e., thermo-receptors in the skin and in the hypothalamus). It sends
information to an integrator that sets the range at which a variable is maintained.

The integrator (i.e., thermo-regulatory centre in the hypothalamus) determines an appropriate response to the stimulus and sends signals to an effector (i.e., vasomotor system, metabolic effectors, sweat glands). After receiving the signal, a change occurs to correct the deviation by enhancing it with feedback mechanisms (Bresjanac and Rupnik 1999). The system works in such a way that deviations between the set point and the measured values are as small as possible. The result is a stable cell environment (Bresjanac and Rupnik 1999). In addition to Maslow, other systems of fundamental human needs and human-scale development exist, such as Manfred Max-Neef's taxonomy of human needs (Manfred et al. 1989), in which needs are positioned without a hierarchy. Human needs in this taxonomy are understood as a system of interrelations and interactivities. Manfred et al. (1989) believed that what changes with time and across cultures is the way that these needs are satisfied.

2.2.2 Overall Comfort

Comfort is defined as: "a state of physical ease and freedom from pain or constraint" (Oxford Dictionaries 2017). **Uncomfortable** conditions are defined as those "not feeling comfortable and pleasant, or not making you feel comfortable and pleasant" (Oxford Dictionaries 2017).

The term "comfort" combines all impact factors that are related to the environmental quality of a healthy building: **thermal comfort, air quality, daylighting, sound comfort, universal design, and ergonomics**. There are constant interactions among parameters of environmental quality factors (Fig. 2.2).

The creation of comfortable conditions for all users is an essential task for building designers as well as system engineers. **"But how can comfortable conditions be achieved in a building?"** One good example of the total achievement of comfortable conditions is a breastfeeding baby in his mother's embrace (Fig. 2.3), which represents a perfect microenvironment in which all the baby's needs are fulfilled: basic physiological needs such as food, water; comfortable thermal environment, optimal level of illumination, the sweet smell and taste of breastmilk, high level of ergonomics, known sounds of the heart beating and breathing, as well as higher needs for love, safety, privacy, and protection. In the same way as the attainment of conditions in the microenvironment for a breastfeeding baby, we have to create conditions inside the active spaces (*medium environment*) of active zones (*macro environment of the whole building*). We have to take into consideration every parameter of overall comfort, with the primary definition of optimal parameters for individual uses.

Several studies have indicated that there are **individual differences in perceptions of comfort**, determined by gender, age, ethnic differences, acclimatization, adaptation, the effect of health status, etc. Moreover, the thermal environment's

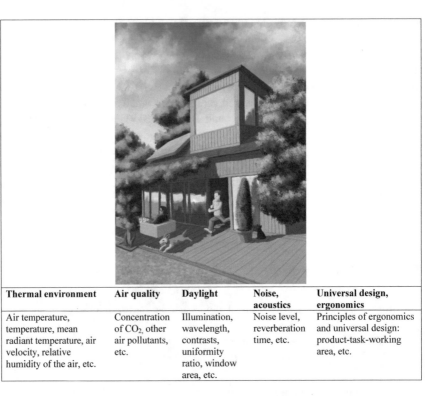

Thermal environment	Air quality	Daylight	Noise, acoustics	Universal design, ergonomics
Air temperature, temperature, mean radiant temperature, air velocity, relative humidity of the air, etc.	Concentration of CO_2, other air pollutants, etc.	Illumination, wavelength, contrasts, uniformity ratio, window area, etc.	Noise level, reverberation time, etc.	Principles of ergonomics and universal design: product-task-working area, etc.

Fig. 2.2 Impact factors and parameters related to the environmental quality of a healthy building

influence on occupants' perceptions of indoor environmental quality depends on various external (i.e., environmental conditions) and internal factors (i.e., user's preferences, experiences, consciousness, etc.). Geng et al. (2017) performed a study on the impact of the **thermal environment** on **occupants' perceptions of indoor environmental quality** (IEQ) and **productivity** in a controlled office under various temperature conditions. The results showed that the variation of the thermal environment not only affected thermal comfort but also had a "comparative" impact on the perception of other IEQ factors. When the thermal environment was unsatisfactory, it weakened the "comfort expectation" of other IEQ factors, which accordingly resulted in less dissatisfaction with other IEQ factors. Conversely, when the thermal environment was quite satisfying, it raised the "**comfort expectation**" of other IEQ factors, which lowered the evaluation of the real performance of other IEQ factors retroactively. In this respect, interactive influences among factors should be considered.

Fig. 2.3 Microenvironment of a breastfeeding baby in mother's embrace

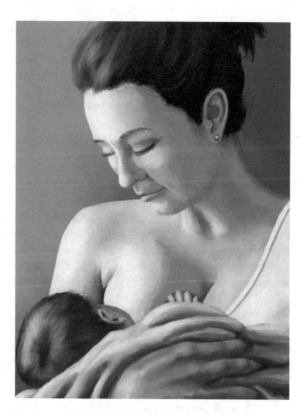

2.2.3 Thermal Comfort

Thermal comfort is described as "a recognizable state of feeling, usually associated with conditions that are pleasant and compatible with health and happiness; and discomfort, with pain which is unpleasant" (Gagge et al. 1967).

According to the definition by the American Society for Heating, Refrigerating and Air-Conditioning Engineers (ASHRAE) (2013), thermal comfort is defined as a "condition of mind that expresses satisfaction with the thermal environment and is assessed by subjective evaluation". *Work on Human Thermal Environments* by Parsons (2014) states that "thermal comfort is a state people strive for when they feel discomfort".

A human being's thermal sensation is influenced by metabolic rate and clothing, as well as the environmental parameters (air temperature, mean radiant temperature, air velocity and air humidity) (ISO 7730: 2005; Fanger 1970), individual characteristics (e.g., gender differences, anthropometric characteristics, cultural differences), and health status (Dovjak et al. 2013; Dovjak 2012; Hwang et al. 2007). A significant effect of gender, age, acclimatization and health status on individual perceptions of thermal comfort conditions has also been proven by studies (Schellen et al. 2010, 2012; Hwang et al. 2007; Karjalainen 2007; Skoog et al. 2005; Parsons 2002; Wallace et al. 1994; Martin et al. 1992; Silverman et al. 1958).

In general environments, **optimal thermal comfort conditions** need to be achieved for the highest possible user satisfaction and productivity (Prek and Butala 2012; Dovjak 2012). Several studies have proved that the optimal thermal environment for the general population and built environments (mainly offices) tends to the slightly cool side of thermal sensation. Lan et al. (2012) proved that such comfortable "cool" environments are beneficial for the performance of office work. Avoiding elevated temperatures in winter and in summer can bring measurable benefits (Lan et al. 2012). Shukuya (2013) and Simone et al. (2011) showed that the minimum **exergy consumption rate** (i.e., the rate of exergy, which is used only for thermoregulation) was associated with thermal sensation votes (TSV) ("vote" in this context means a point of time when a human subject filled out a thermal sensation scale during exposure) close to thermal neutrality but tending to the slightly cool side of thermal sensation.

Furthermore, in the general environment and population, there are significant variations in thermal acceptance between individuals. A quantitative interview survey with a total of 3,094 respondents in Finland showed significant gender differences in thermal comfort and temperature preference. Females are less satisfied with room temperatures than males are, prefer higher room temperatures than males do, and feel both uncomfortably cold and uncomfortably hot more often than males do. Although females are more critical of their thermal environments, males use thermostats in households more often than females do (Karjalainen 2007; Schellen et al. 2012). However, several studies also indicate that the thermal neutral temperature and optimum thermal condition differ between young adults and the elderly. Schellen et al. (2010) concluded that the elderly preferred a higher temperature in comparison to young adults.

In reality, designers are often confronted with the highly demanding task of designing conditions for specific environments, such as **hospitals**, which are a complex environment that can be treated as a three-dimensional system of specific users (patients, staff, visitors), as well as specific activity and active spaces. In active spaces, the required conditions for patients need to support medical treatment and result in quicker recovery and positive health outcomes. Immediately after the definition of specific user needs for comfort conditions, the building systems that enable creating those conditions have to be defined.

User diversity is the main guidance when designing buildings, and systems. In most cases, conventional HVAC systems are designed as interventions in active spaces, based on the requirements of an average user and are not suitable for the selected individual user. Dovjak (2012) concluded, "to fulfil specific individual requirements, new systems are needed". Individual climates have already been introduced in cars. Local ventilation is used in working environments with a positive impact on productivity (Melikov et al. 2002). Overall individualization of personal space that would enable **individual generation and control of all factors of environmental ergonomics** has been implemented in a test environment by the research group of Dovjak and colleagues (Dovjak et al. 2013, 2014; Dovjak 2012).

The innovative system creates optimal conditions for health care and treatment of burn patients with lower human body exergy consumption rates, valid for thermoregulation, minimal evaporation, radiation, and convection. For health care workers and visitors, the low exergy (LowEx) system (i.e., heating-cooling ceiling radiative panels) creates individual thermal comfort zones by allowing the setting of air temperature and mean radiant temperature. For the LowEx system, the measured energy use for heating was 11–27% lower and for cooling 32–73% lower than for conventional systems (Dovjak et al. 2013, 2014; Dovjak 2012).

Improving comfort has to be one of the main drives for renovations and not just saving energy. Interestingly, users are aware of these issues. Velux (2017), a series of Pan-European surveys, determined that renovation, mainly due to increased comfort conditions and health, is one of the leading motives of occupants. Moreover, not only for renovation, but Europeans also value comfort the most when choosing a new home.

2.3   Wellbeing and Sustainable Buildings

As part of the definition renewal efforts in 1948, the term health was associated with the high level of **well-being** (wellbeing, or wellness) (WHO 1986).

> High level of well-being is described as a dynamic process in which the individual is actively engaged in moving toward fulfilment of his or her potential (Medical Dictionary 2017).

Wellness refers to diverse and interconnected dimensions of physical, mental, and social well-being that extend beyond the traditional definition of health. It includes choices and activities aimed at achieving physical vitality, mental alacrity, social satisfaction, a sense of accomplishment, and personal fulfilment (Naci and Ioannidis 2015). It means in some sense the individual or group's condition is positive.

There exist several models of wellbeing. Diener's tripartite model of subjective well-being is one of the most comprehensive models of well-being in psychology (Tov and Diener 2013). Carol Ryff's multidimensional model of **psychological well-being** (Ryff and Keyes 1995) postulated six factors that are key to well-being:

- Autonomy
- Environmental Mastery
- Personal Growth
- Positive Relations with Others
- Purpose in Life
- Self-Acceptance.

In Carol Ryff's model, wellbeing is quantitatively evaluated by a series of statements reflecting the six areas of psychological well-being. Respondents rate statements on a scale of 1–6, with 1 indicating strong disagreement and 6 indicating strong agreement. For each category, a high score indicates that the respondent has a mastery of that area in his or her life. High scores indicate that the respondent makes effective use of opportunities and has a sense of mastery in managing environmental factors and activities, including managing everyday affairs and creating situations to benefit personal needs (Ryff and Keyes 1995).

> An example statement for environmental mastery is: "In general, I feel I am in charge of the situation in which I live" (Ryff and Keyes 1995).

The five-item **WHO Well-Being Index (WHO-5)** is among the most widely used questionnaires assessing subjective psychological well-being. Since its first publication in 1998, the WHO-5 has been translated into more than 30 languages and has been used in research studies all over the world (Topp et al. 2015). The WHO-5 is a short questionnaire consisting of five simple and non-invasive questions, which tap into the subjective well-being of the respondents. The WHO-5 items are (Topp et al. 2015):

(Q1) "I have **felt cheerful and in good** spirits",
(Q2) "I have **felt calm and relaxed**",
(Q3) "I have **felt active and vigorous**",
(Q4) "I woke up **feeling fresh and rested**" and
(Q5) "My daily life has been filled with **things that interest me**"

We can note that the quality of built environments affects the subjective well-being and the quality of our lives. As people age, their quality of life is largely determined by their ability to maintain autonomy and independence (Public Health England 2016; WHO 2002). **"Do the conditions in current buildings allow us to attain wellbeing of an individual or a group?"** Supporters of popularized sustainable design, eco-friendly, green and low carbon architecture claim that their building practices expand and complement the classical building design concerns of economy, utility, durability, and comfort (EPA 2009).

> **Quality of life** is "an individual's perception of his or her position in life in the context of the culture and value system where they live, and in relation to their goals, expectations, standards and concerns. It is a broad ranging concept, incorporating in a complex way a person's physical health, psychological state, level of independence, social relationships, personal beliefs and relationship to salient features in the environment" (WHO 2017b, p. 1).

2.3.1 Sustainable, Eco-friendly, Green and Low Carbon Buildings

The term **harmonized, nature-oriented (ecological) development** was defined by the Council of Europe in 1966. It stands for a development in one direction, within a specific area. For example, economic development indicates a process of development of a country or region in the direction of increasing wealth in order to achieve the well-being of the population. The verb *to sustain* means "to maintain; keep in existence; keep going; prolong" (Bossel 1999). The term **sustainable development** was defined by the Brundtland Report in 1987 and by the UN Conference on Environment and Development in Rio de Janeiro in 1992 (WCED 1987; Rio Declaration 1992).

> *Sustainable development means the development where all four aspects are equally balanced: health, environmental, social and economic* (Rio Declaration 1992).

The World Commission on Environment and Development (WCED) (1987) states that sustainable development is "a development that meets the needs of the present without compromising the ability of future generations to meet their own needs". Therefore, it provides all the inhabitants of the planet appropriate quality of life. Sustainable development of human society has environmental, material, ecological, social, economic, legal, cultural, political and psychological dimensions that require attention (Bossel 1999). Their mutual interactions are emphasized in the framework of Environmental Impact Assessment (EIA) defined by Directive 2011/92/EU (Directive 2011/92/EU, Directive 2001/42/EC). **Sustainability** is a dynamic concept and involves a time dimension (Bossel 1999).

Nowadays, the term is often **popularized** and **exploited**, especially in the building sector. Generally, incorrect definitions are in use, where only one aspect of development is well considered, while others are ignored. Examples of buildings and their negative consequences on health were presented in Chap. 1.

Moreover, controversies exist among environmentalists who argue that sustainable development was formulated by economists, as an environmentally friendly capitalism, in order to pacify people and to promote environmental values. Consequently, it is necessary to understand that for humans the environment is irrelevant if one is not part of it as an active element that lives and works in it. An equitable, environmentally and physically sustainable society that exploits the environment at the highest sustainable rate would still be psychologically and culturally unsustainable. **Unsustainability** is one alternative to **sustainability** (Bossel 1999). **Unsustainable activities** are all human activities that have a negative impact on the environment and health. If it is assessed, for any human activity, that it is unsustainable, it should be abstained from and not performed (EC 1992).

Currently, several **building certification schemes** to measure the sustainability of the buildings (Ding 2008) exist: Leadership in Energy and Environmental Design (LEED), Research Establishment Environment Assessment Methodology (BREEAM), Deutsche Gesellschaft für Nachhaltiges Bauen (DGNB), Haute Qualité Environnementale (HQE), etc. These tools audit selected criteria, which score the investigated parameter and sum up and weight the partial scores to arrive at the final score that evaluates the sustainability of a building (Potrč et al. 2017). The parameters can be quantitative, and the score is obtained based on the quantitative result for a parameter. Qualitative parameters are most often assessed based on criteria that determine whether a certain standard is achieved or not (Forsberg and von Malmborg 2004).

The existing sustainable **building certification schemes** already include selected aspects related to **comfort, well-being, and productivity** of occupants. For example, air quality, water quality, visual and overall comfort (mostly related to thermal and acoustic comfort), are topics well covered in LEED, DGNB, BREEM. **Mind** (assessing parameters influencing the mental state of the occupants), **fitness** (assessing parameters connected to the increase of physical activity of the occupants), and **nourishment** (accessing parameters related to the fresh, wholesome food) are not covered in the existing certification schemes (Potrč et al. 2017). Currently, a **specialized certification scheme** called **WELL**, launched by The International Well Building Institute in 2014, focuses on the assessment of **health- and well-being-related questions in the built environment** (WELL 2016). A similar certification program is the **Living Building Challenge**, created by the International Living Future Institute in 2006 (Living Building Challenge 2017). Other tools that evaluate the sustainability of a building are **Health, Wellbeing and Productivity in Offices** published by the World Green Building Council (WGBC 2014) and **FitWell launched** by the Center for Active Design (Fitwel 2016).

Based on established knowledge, Potrč et al. (2017) performed a comparative analysis of the existing building certification schemes on health aspects. Potrč and colleagues (2017) concluded that the WELL building certification scheme can be used as a complementary scheme that supports the existing building certification schemes. Some of the topics are duplicated, but generally, the WELL certification scheme focuses only on the aspects connected to health and wellbeing while other certification schemes put greater emphasis on other aspects.

Additionally, Markelj et al. (2014) highlighted that current tools and methods are either focused only on individual topics or are too complex and not adapted to independent use by architects. They proposed a simplified method for evaluating building sustainability that can be used in the early design phase. The use of building certification schemes is not required. Many of the investors decide to perform a certification to show their awareness and to gain a better insight into the performance of their buildings (Potrč et al. 2017).

The term "**green architecture**" only came into use in the 1990s (The Economist 2004), but the movement's roots can be traced back a long way. Crystal Palace in Hyde Park, London, designed by Joseph Paxton (Crystal Palace 2008), and Milan's Galleria Vittorio Emanuele II designed by Giuseppe Mengoni (Milan 2012), for example, built in 1851 and 1877 respectively, used roof ventilators and underground air-cooling chambers to regulate the indoor temperature. Green building (also known as green construction or sustainable building) has a similar approach as eco-friendly building and refers to both a structure and the application of processes that are **environmentally responsible** and **resource-efficient** throughout a building's life-cycle: from planning to design, construction, operation, maintenance, renovation, and demolition (EPA 2009). LEED (Leadership in Energy and Environmental Design) developed by the **U.S. Green Building Council** is a building certification scheme for the design, construction, operation, and maintenance of green buildings (EPA 2009).

> *Eco-friendly building or ecological construction is building a structure that is beneficial or non-harmful to the environment, and resource efficient. This type of construction is efficient in its use of local and renewable materials, and in the energy required to build it, and the energy generated while being within it* (SustainableBuild 2017).

Due to legal requirements towards low carbon economy, low-carbon design emerged. Low-carbon buildings are buildings designed and constructed to release very little or no carbon at all during their lifetime. They are designed according to the standard Low-Carbon Buildings Method TM 2011, Buildings Construction, A Simplified Methodology for Estimating GHG Emissions from Buildings Construction. They are specifically engineered with greenhouse gases reduction in mind.

> *A **low-carbon building** is a building that emits significantly fewer greenhouse gases than regular buildings.*

The existing movement towards **eco-building**, **sustainable building**, **low-carbon building**, and **green building** has been used in many studies, especially in engineering. However, these studies cannot represent the health status of buildings comprehensively and appropriately (Mao et al. 2017).

What is required to make all those energy efficient buildings healthy? In the field of building design, many legal acts and standards that separately cover issues related to energy, environment or comfort exist. When all those requirements and recommendations are combined in the design process, they might be even contradictory. Moreover, current certification schemes are often not mandatory and performed after the decision has been made by investors. For the design of healthy and sustainable buildings, an integral certification system that combines existing "energy and environmental" schemes with "health and wellbeing schemes" are needed.

The passive house standard (IPHA 2018) defines criteria for the certification of passive building: space heating and cooling requirements, primary energy requirements, airtightness, and thermal comfort. Although the current standard stands for quality, comfort and energy efficiency in general buildings, the qualitative and quantitative criteria for indoor environmental quality, namely indoor air quality, daylighting, and noise issues are defined insufficiently, especially in relation to a building, system, and user characteristics. The defined criteria are presented as minimal values, which often results in insufficient indoor environmental conditions. Therefore, the design of overall comfort conditions in current practice often depends on the designer's and/or investor's awareness. Moreover, especially energy use and indoor quality issues are also related to user behaviour (Schweiker et al. 2018), and they might be changed as soon as the building is used. Designed values might not result in proper indoor air quality, so it is important to raise the awareness of building occupants how to change or regulate building and its systems.

The WELL Building Standard (WELL 2016) focuses solely on the health and wellness of building occupants. It identifies 100 performance metrics, design strategies, and policies that can be implemented by the owners, designers, engineers, contractors, users, and operators of a building. WELL certification can be applied to new and existing buildings (i.e., commercial, institutional), building interiors as well as core and shell. The WELL Building Standard is organized into seven categories of wellness called concepts: air, water, nourishment, light, fitness, comfort and mind. Every feature is ascribed to human body systems (e.g., cardiovascular, digestive, endocrine systems) and is intended to address specific aspects of occupant health, comfort, or knowledge. Projects become certified on the basis of the dynamic rating system, according to the number of features that are sufficiently satisfied. The final WELL Score is calculated based on the total preconditions and optimizations achieved across the board—not as a function of averaging independent concept scores. To maintain WELL certification, projects must be recertified a minimum of every three years, because building conditions can deteriorate over time to the point of adversely affecting the health and wellness of occupants. The WELL protocol requires highly qualified assessor (WELL 2016).

The design of a healthy buildings is a highly demanding process that requires participatory design, in which all stakeholders including end users are actively involved. Regarding the fact that health issues are unsystematically and insufficiently covered in the existing sustainability building standards, they might be complemented with the concepts presented in the WELL Building Standard. Although the main advantage of the existing WELL Building Standard is its comprehensiveness, it can be upgraded by more systematic classification of the health and wellbeing concepts.

2.4 Health Effects in the Built Environment

Because of the busy pace of modern life—performing daily activities related to work, commuting, taking care of kids, cooking and cleaning, watching television, connecting on social media, and more—people are spending most of the day indoors.

The National Human Activity Pattern Survey (NHAPS) performed a two-year probability-based telephone survey (N = 9,386) of exposure-related human activities in the United States sponsored by the U.S. Environmental Protection Agency (EPA) (Klepeis et al. 2001). The results of the survey (total sample N = 9.196) showed that respondents spent 68.7% of the time in a residence, 5.4% in an office or factory, 1.8% in a bar or restaurant, 11% in some other indoor location. The total time spent indoors was 86.9%; 5.5% of the time was spent in a vehicle and 7.6% outdoors. These results are comparable with U.S. time-budgets reported by Robinson and Thomas (1991) from a 1985 study and Canadian time budgets reported by Leech et al. (1996). For both these studies, which span a period of about a decade, respondents reported spending 89% of their time indoors with 5% in a vehicle and 6% outdoors. Smith (1993) showed that the differences between developed and less-developed countries, and urban and rural environments. The percentage of time spent indoors in less developed countries was 79% for urban environments and 65% for rural environments. The percentage of time spent outdoors in less developed countries was 21% for urban environments and 35% for rural environments (Smith 1993).

According to the report of the European Commission, Directorate General for Health and Consumers (Jantunen et al. 2011) and the EC (2007), people spend 60–90% of their lives in indoor environments. Ribble Cycles surveyed (2017) more than a thousand adults in Britain, finding that the average person spent 92% of their time indoors on a weekly basis. However, vulnerable groups of people, such as the elderly, immobile persons, patients etc., spend even more time indoors. Most children spend approximately one fourth of the day in day-care centres, schools, and other educational institutions. The National Kids Survey determined that after school they prefer to choose technology-centred activities than nature-based activities (Larson et al. 2011). Data from the National Kids Survey by Larson et al. (2011) (N = 1,450 U.S. households with children ages 6–19, from 2007 to 2009) showed that, in general, most children (>62.5%) spent at least two hours of time outdoors daily. Similar conclusions were made in a National Trust survey (N = 1,001 parents with children aged between four and 14), in which researchers found, on average, children were playing outside for just over four hours a week, compared to 8.2 h a week when the adults questioned were children (The Guardian 2016).

During the time spend inside built environments we are exposed to numerous environmental hazards.

> An **environmental hazard** is a substance, state or event that has the potential to threaten the surrounding natural environment and/or adversely affect people's health.

A number of systems used to characterize environmental hazards exists (Stevens and Hall 1993). According to the book "Basic Environmental Health" by Yassi et al. (2001), environmental hazards are most commonly classified as either:

- biological,
- chemical,
- physical,
- biomechanical, and
- psychosocial.

Exposure to these hazards can affect human health. The extent of the effects is dependent on their exposure dose, type of pollutants, exposure time, and individual characteristics (Eržen et al. 2010; Yassi et al. 2001). Poor indoor environmental quality conditions (i.e., thermal discomfort, inadequate air quality, noise, lack of daylight, electromagnetic radiation, etc.), longer exposure times, the presence of vulnerable population groups, and increased user susceptibility may increase the risk of adverse health effects. **Health effects (or health impacts)** are changes in health resulting from exposure to a source.

Health effects resulting from exposure to a source in a built environment should be an important topic not only for environmental public health but also for the engineering sciences. The prevention of health effects in the built environment is the main activity in every step of design. In a review by Lavin et al. (2006), many health impacts in built environments were defined according to the type of health hazard (i.e., radon, environmental tobacco smoke, cooking pollutants, volatile organic compounds, asbestos). The most common health outcome in research studies and public media is **Sick Building Syndrome (SBS)**. Sick Building Syndrome is often confused with **Building-Related Illness (BRI)**. Therefore, for further understanding, it is important to distinguish between them.

2.4.1   Sick Building Syndrome Versus Building-Related Illness

The US Environmental Protection Agency (EPA 1991) describes **Sick Building Syndrome (SBS)** as situations in which building occupants experience acute health and comfort effects that appear to be linked to time spent in a building, but no specific illness or cause can be identified. The complaints may be localized in a particular room or zone or may be widespread throughout the building. The characteristic symptoms of SBS that may occur singly or in combination with each other are headache, eye, nose, or throat irritation, dry cough, dry or itchy skin, dizziness and nausea, difficulty in concentrating, fatigue and sensitivity to odours (Redlich et al. 1997; ECA 1989; Burge et al. 1987). In contrast, the term **Building-Related Illness (BRI)** is used when symptoms of a diagnosable illness are identified and can be attributed directly to airborne building contaminants (EPA 1991). SBS does not include diseases caused by exposure to a specific cause in the environment (e.g., mould, spores or allergens) (Redlich et al. 1997). The main differences between SBS and BRI are presented in Table 2.1.

The syndrome first appeared in the 1970s with the development of energy-efficient buildings equipped with mechanical systems for heating, ventilation, and air-conditioning (HVAC). Some of the possible causes are the use of synthetic building materials, overcrowded workplaces, and stress in the workplace. Currently, none of the environmental factors has been identified as the sole cause of SBS, and the latter is likely to be a common consequence of biological, chemical and organic agents, as well as personal and individual factors (Redlich et al. 1997).

Table 2.1 Differences between Sick Building Syndromesick building syndrom (SBS) and Building-Related Illness (BRI) (Burge 2004; Redlich et al.1997; EPA 1991)

Indicators	Description	
	SBS	BRI
Symptomatology	Building occupants complain of symptoms associated with acute discomfort, e.g., headache; eye, nose, or throat irritation; dry cough; dry or itchy skin; dizziness and nausea; difficulty in concentrating; fatigue; and sensitivity to odours	Building occupants complain of symptoms, such as cough; chest tightness; fever, chills; and muscle aches
Diagnosis	Non-diagnosable illness	Diagnosable illness
Aetiology (cause)	The cause of the symptoms is not known	The symptoms can be clinically defined and have clearly identifiable causes
Duration	Most complainants report relief soon after leaving the building	Complainants may require prolonged recovery times after leaving the building

Approximately 30% of new and renovated buildings worldwide may be affected by SBS (WHO 1983).

SBS symptoms may occur in residential and public buildings (Sahlberg et al. 2013; Takigawa et al. 2012; Araki et al. 2010; Engvall et al. 2001; Scheel et al. 2001). In studies on residential buildings in Japan (N = 871, Takigawa et al. 2012; N = 620, Araki et al. 2010), and residential buildings in three northern European cities (N = 159, Sahlberg et al. 2013), from 12% to 30.8% of occupants were identified as having SBS symptoms. Moreover, in the studies on public buildings in Canada (N = 1,390, Bourbeau et al. 1997), UK (N = 4.373, Burge et al. 1987), USA (N = 600, Woods et al. 1987) from 20% to 50% of workers experienced SBS symptoms.

A comprehensive study (Burge et al. 1987) performed in the UK on 4,373 office workers in 42 public buildings revealed that 29% of those studied experienced five or more of the characteristic SBS symptoms. An investigation carried out by Woods et al. (1987) on 600 office workers in the US concluded that 20% of the employees experienced SBS symptoms and most of them were convinced that this reduced their working efficiency. Additionally, a study on 1,390 workers in 5 public buildings in Quebec, Canada (Bourbeau et al. 1997) showed that 50% of workers experienced SBS symptoms. Moreover, much higher prevalence of SBS was demonstrated in hospital environment than in other public buildings. A review study by Kalender Smajlović et al. (2019) found that the prevalence of SBS was from 41% to 87%.

SBS is characterized by "**non-specific symptoms**, occurring while living/ working in the building and not causing a specific disease or infection. Due to individual differences and non-specific symptoms, some experts do not define SBS as an independent syndrome. Currently there exist more than 50 possible symptoms of SBS that appear in different combinations and strengths" (Burge 2004, p. 185, Redlich et al. 1997, p. 1013).

In general, we divide symptoms into five groups (ECA 1989):

- **Nasal manifestations**: nasal irritation, rhinorrhoea, nasal obstruction
- **Ocular manifestations**: dryness and irritation of the mucous membrane of the eye
- **Oropharyngeal manifestations**: dryness and irritation of the throat
- **Cutaneous manifestations**: dryness and irritation of the skin, occasionally associated with a rash on exposed skin surfaces
- **General manifestations**: headaches and generalized lethargy and tiredness leading to poor concentration.

Unlike **SBS**, **BRI** is usually grouped into four groups (ECA 1989):

- Allergy, asthma, rhinitis
- Hypersensitivity pneumonitis (extrinsic allergic alveolitis)
- Humidifier fever
- Infections (bacterial, fungal, viral).

2.5 Health Outcomes Related to Unhealthy Built Environments

> **Health outcomes** are "a change in the health status of an individual, group or population which is attributable to a planned intervention or series of interventions, regardless of whether such an intervention was intended to change health status" (WHO 1998, p. 10).

Findings from the relevant epidemiological studies and reports are mainly focused on European populations and are presented later in this book. A Pan-European study, Velux (2015) (N = 12,000, October 2014), demonstrated a clear correlation between unhealthy buildings and people who have rated the parameter of self-perceived health as "poor". Today, one out of six Europeans—or the equivalent of Germany's population—reports living in unhealthy buildings. More than one-and-a-half times as many people who live in unhealthy buildings have poor health compared to those who live in healthy buildings.

The most common indicators of inadequate indoor environments are (Velux 2015):

- building **dampness**,
- poor indoor **air quality**,
- **uncomfortable thermal** environment,
- excessive **noise**, and
- lack of **daylight**.

In addition, safety, space, accessibility, location, and immediate surroundings are significant influences of the internal environment (Lavin et al. 2006). They cause or affect health outcomes and result in diseases and injuries, such as respiratory, nervous system and cardiovascular diseases, and cancer (WHO 1992).

Global Health Observatory (GHO) data (WHO 2017c) revealed that in 2012, **12.6 million people died as a result of living or working in an unhealthy environment**, representing 23% of all deaths. When accounting for both death and disability, the fraction of the global burden of disease due to the environment is 22%. In children under five years, up to 26% of all deaths could be prevented, if environmental risks were removed. For effective interventions, all indicators of inadequate indoor environments must be eliminated. In the following subchapters, (Sects. 2.5.1 to 2.5.5), the most important ones will be more precisely defined.

2.5.1 Building Dampness

One of the most common indicators of an inadequate indoor environment is **building dampness**.

> The term **building dampness** includes: "the increased indoor air humidity and/or damp construction complexes that often results in mould growth" (WHO 2009a; p. 2, Kukec et al. 2015, p. 36).

Building dampness most frequently results from **inadequate ventilation, improper design of the building envelope and systems, inadequate damp-proof membrane, damaged plumbing systems, floods, occupants' habits, and the position of furniture**. In addition to inequalities in building and system design, activities and occupant behaviour are significant causes of dampness. Velux (2015) showed that 65% of all Europeans dry clothes indoors at least once a week, and only 28% ventilate rooms more than once a day during winter, which is needed to obtain optimal indoor air quality.

Building dampness in the indoor built environment may constitute a substandard living and working condition. It indicates the presence of water damage, a leaking roof, rot in window frames and floors, visible mould or condensation. Building dampness is associated with a broad array of detrimental health effects in adults and children (Fisk et al. 2010). The most common of these are related to the deterioration of the respiratory system (Mudarri and Fisk 2007), including a higher prevalence of respiratory symptoms, increased risk of asthma, wheezing, cough (Pirastu et al. 2009), bronchitis, common cold and rhinitis (Pirhonen et al. 1996).

Epidemiologic studies and cost-effect analysis in the US and the EU have revealed that building dampness has a substantial **public health and economic impact** (Fisk et al. 2010). Researchers from the U.S. Department of Energy's Lawrence Berkeley National Laboratory (Berkeley Lab), concluded that building dampness and mould raised the risk of a variety of respiratory and asthma-related health outcomes in the U.S. by 30–50%. The public health and economic impact of dampness and mould was assessed by Mudarri and Fisk (2007), who determined that of the 21.8 million people reported to have asthma in the U.S., approximately 4.6 million cases are estimated to be attributable to dampness and mould exposure at home. They estimated that in the US national annual cost of asthma that is attributable to dampness and mould exposure at home was $3.5 billion (Mudarri and Fisk 2007).

A pan-European study, Velux (2015) (N = 12,000, October 2014), revealed that **80 million Europeans live in damp and unhealthy buildings**, which nearly doubles the risk of developing asthma. The cost to European societies of asthma and chronic obstructive pulmonary disease is €82 billion per year (Velux 2017). In fact, people are 40% more likely to have asthma when living in a damp or mouldy home, and today, 2.2 million Europeans have asthma as a result of their living conditions. Half of that amount goes to direct costs such as medicine and care. The other half is calculated as indirect costs due to loss of work productivity (Velux 2017).

2.5.2   Uncomfortable Thermal Environment

Uncomfortable thermal environment in a building is directly related to the building and systems efficiency on the specific location. Additionally, family income plays a key role in ensuring a comfortable thermal environment. This means that household's ability to keep the home adequately warm or cold is dependent on the indicator of fuel poverty (a person is to be regarded as living "in fuel poverty" if he is a member of a household living on a lower income in a home which cannot be kept warm at reasonable cost) (WHECA 2000). In Europe, between 50 and 125 million people are estimated to suffer from fuel poverty and the Epee Project reveals that this number will inevitably rise in the future as global energy prices increase (BPIE 2014).

It is important to recognize that a **household's inability** to keep the home adequately warm or cold has serious health consequences. In a European cross-country analysis (Healy 2003), a statistically significant association between poor housing thermal efficiency and high levels of winter mortality was found. According to the recent Marmot Review Team report (2011) on the health impacts of cold housing and fuel poverty, excess winter deaths (EWDs) in England, are associated with thermal efficiency of housing and low indoor temperatures. About 40% and 33% of excess winter deaths are attributable to cardiovascular and respiratory diseases respectively, the risk of excess winter death being almost three times higher in the quartile of houses with the coldest indoor temperatures than in the warmest quartile. European studies on the burden of disease of inadequate housing quantified as 30% the proportion of excess winter deaths attributable to cold housing (Braubach et al. 2011). Results of the pan-European study, Velux (2017) showed that forty-five percent of people keep their temperatures down in order to lower their energy bills. Twice as many Europeans report poor health when they are unable to keep their dwelling at a comfortable temperature in the winter; 20% of Europeans report poor health when they are living in cold home, and 9% of Europeans report poor health when they are living in a comfortably warm home.

Climate change is expected to cause increases in heat-related mortality, especially from respiratory and cardiovascular diseases (Basagaña et al. 2011). Children and the elderly are the most vulnerable groups. The effects of heat on morbidity across all age groups and across a wider range of temperatures in Rhode Island were clarified by Kingsley et al. (2016). Their findings suggest that the current population of Rhode Island would experience substantially higher morbidity and mortality if maximum daily temperatures increase further as projected.

2.5.3 Poor Indoor Air Quality

Indoor air is often more seriously polluted than outdoor air even in the largest and most industrialized cities (EPA 2017). Indoor air may contain over 900 chemicals, particles and biological materials with potential health effects (EC 2007).

Problems of indoor air quality are recognized as important risk factors for human health in low-, middle- and high-income countries. WHO (2016) reported:

- **Globally, 4.3 million people a year die** from exposure to household air pollution.
- Over **4 million people die prematurely** from illness attributable to the household air pollution from cooking with solid fuels.
- More than **50% of premature deaths** due to pneumonia among children under 5 are caused by particulate matter (soot) inhaled from household air pollution.
- **3.8 million premature deaths** annually from noncommunicable diseases including stroke, ischaemic heart disease, chronic obstructive pulmonary disease (COPD) and lung cancer are attributed to exposure to household air pollution.

Hazardous substances emitted from buildings, construction materials and indoor equipment or due to human activities indoors, such as combustion of fuels for cooking or heating, lead to a broad range of health problems and may even be fatal. World Health Organization (WHO 2010) identified five important hazardous substances which have been linked to respiratory diseases including asthma, lung cancer and mesothelioma by the:

- radon
- environmental tobacco smoke (ETS)
- cooking pollutants
- volatile organic compounds and
- asbestos.

A pan-European study, Velux (2015) revealed that unhealthy indoor air quality is a concern for Europeans; 24% of Europeans are very concerned, and 59% have above average concern. They rank this concern at the same level as financial and job insecurity. A total of 35% of Europeans rank both indoor air quality of the highest importance if moving to a new house. If they were to choose a new home, 42% would give the highest importance to the indoor air; 89% would give it above average importance, resulting in an indicator score of 6. A total of 28% have made changes within the last five years to improve indoor air quality. Moreover, 55% of

Europeans aged 60 to 65 assign indoor air quality the highest importance, compared to 31% of the 18–29-year olds.

2.5.4   Excessive Noise

Noise pollution is considered not only an environmental nuisance but also a threat to public health (WHO 2011). In indoor environments, we are exposed to numerous noise sources emitted from outdoor to indoor environments. Sound protection of buildings provides protection against the following sources of noise:

- **external noise** (e.g., traffic noise, noise from industrial facilities),
- **airborne noise** (i.e., transmitted by air and atmosphere),
- **structure-borne noise** from other spaces (i.e., transmitted when sound arises from the impact of an object on a building element such as a wall, floor, or ceiling),
- **noise of operating equipment** (e.g., HVAC), and
- **reverberation noise** (i.e., collection of reflected sounds from the surfaces in an enclosure).

The results of the classification of buildings by sound protection in the EU show that the large majority of the buildings are classified into Class D (poor sound insulation of the building envelope, internal constructional complexes) (Rasmussen 2010). Inadequate sound protection of buildings consequently results in increased occupant exposure. Epidemiological studies indicate that those chronically exposed to high levels of environmental noise have an increased risk of cardiovascular diseases, such as myocardial infarction. The evidence from epidemiological studies on the association between exposure to road traffic and aircraft noise and hypertension and ischaemic heart disease has increased in recent years. Night-time noise is thought to be particularly problematic as it can affect sleep with subsequent impacts on health (WHO 2009b).

One of the negative effects of exposure to noise is **tinnitus** (i.e., the sensation of sound in the absence of an external sound source). In some people, tinnitus can cause sleep disturbance, cognitive effects, anxiety, psychological distress, depression, communication problems, frustration, irritability, tension, inability to work, reduced efficiency and restricted participation in social life. Globally, tinnitus caused by excessive noise exposure has long been described; 50–90% of patients with chronic noise trauma report tinnitus (WHO 2011).

To estimate the environmental burden of disease (EBD) due to environmental noise, a quantitative risk assessment was performed by WHO (2011). The EBD is expressed as disability-adjusted life years (DALYs). DALYs are the sum of the potential years of life lost due to premature death and the equivalent years of "healthy" life lost by virtue of being in states of poor health or disability. The burden of disease due to environmental noise has been recently estimated for western European countries with a range of 1.0–1.6 million DALYs lost across all health outcomes (WHO 2011). The estimates are 61,000 DALYs for ischaemic heart disease, 45,000 for cognitive impairment of children, 903,000 for sleep disturbance, 22,000 for tinnitus, and 587,000 for annoyance.

> Exposure to noise in living and working environments might cause both auditory and non-auditory adverse health effects (Basner et al. 2014).

Adverse effects of noise on the human body depend on sound intensity, frequency, impulsiveness, duration of exposure (acute, chronic) and the individual's sensitivity. Impairment might be temporary or permanent and is a result of cumulative effects of noise exposure over the course of a lifetime.

Noise-induced hearing loss can be caused by a one-time exposure to an intense impulse sound, or by steady long-term exposure with sound pressure levels higher than 75–85 dB, in occupational and industrial settings. Hearing loss is increasingly caused by social noise exposure (Basner et al. 2014).

A review study by Basner et al. (2014) found that the non-auditory effects of environmental noise exposure on public health are growing. The most investigated non-auditory health endpoints for noise exposure are perceived disturbance and annoyance, cognitive impairment (mainly in children), sleep disturbance, and cardiovascular health (Basner et al. 2014). They can be caused by an exposure with lower sound pressure levels compared to levels that caused auditory adverse health effects. For example, maximum sound pressure levels as low as 33 dB can induce physiological reactions during sleep including autonomic, motor, and cortical arousals (e.g., tachycardia, body movements, and awakenings) (WHO 2009b). Additionally, infrasound might have adverse health effects. Jeffery (2013) highlighted that people who live or work in proximity to industrial wind turbines have experienced symptoms that include decreased quality of life, annoyance, stress, sleep disturbance, headache, anxiety, depression, and cognitive dysfunction. Causes of symptoms include a combination of wind turbine noise, infrasound, electricity, ground current, and shadow flicker. Environmental noise exposure must be regulated by holistic actions, including sound prevention measures in buildings.

Beside building dampness and noise, lack of daylight also contributes to the inadequate environmental quality of the built environment.

2.5.5 Lack of Daylight

Positive influences of daylighting on well-being have been researched since the 1950s.

Daylighting in a built environment has two important effects on the human body: *visual and non-visual* (Robbins 1986; Berson et al. 2002)

Fist studies were concerned with visual effects (i.e., reduced eyestrain) (Robbins 1986) and the psychological benefits of daylight (i.e., improved mood) (Heerwagen 1986). The physiological mechanisms of non-visual effects were fully explained with the discovery of the third photoreceptor cells by David Berson (Berson et al. 2002). Since 2002, studies have been focused mainly on non-visual effects of daylight, which include direct or non-circadian effects, indirect or circadian effects, effects on skin (vitamin D synthesis, skin tanning, and dissociation of bilirubin) and other unexplored effects. Current studies demonstrate the positive impact of daylight in office environments, educational institutions, retail environments, health-care facilities, and in prisons. In addition to **health benefits**, daylight in built environments also has **social, economic** and **environmental benefits**. The social benefits have been associated with improved mood and enhanced morale (Robbins 1986), increased social interactions among employees, and reduced absenteeism rates (Clark and Watson 1988). The economic benefits of daylighting were analysed especially in office environments and were increased productivity. The environmental benefits of daylighting include lower CO_2 emissions and annual energy savings for lighting due to changes in a typical six-storey office building (Jenkins and Newborough 2007).

A lack of daylight in built environments has adverse health effects on human health and their determinants. One of them presents **Seasonal Affective Disorder (SAD)**.

SAD characterized by "fall/winter major depression with spring/summer remission, is a prevalent mental health problem. SAD etiology is not certain, but available models focus on neurotransmitters, hormones, circadian rhythm dysregulation, genetic polymorphisms, and psychological factors" (Roecklein and Rohan 2005, p. 20).

SAD has a seasonal pattern, usually beginning in fall and continuing into the winter months. Those who live in northern latitudes are most at risk. An estimated 10–20% of recurrent depression cases follow a seasonal pattern (Magnusson 2000). Although a summer pattern of recurrence is possible, the predominant pattern involves fall/winter depression with spring/summer remission. In U.S. community surveys, SAD prevalence ranges from 9.7% in New Hampshire to 1.4% in Florida (Rosen et al. 1990). In North America, SAD prevalence increases with latitude, but the correlation is nonsignificant in other parts of the world (Mersch et al. 1999). In the United Kingdom, 20% experience "winter blues" and 2% experience SAD (UK SAD). Light therapy is established as the best available treatment for SAD

(Roecklein and Rohan 2005). A study by Espiritu et al. (1994) on 104 subjects aged 40–64 years in San Diego, CA. The median subject was exposed to illumination greater than or equal to 1000 lux for only 4% of the time observed, that is, only about 58 min per day were spent in daylight. Exposure to that amount of daylight does not provide adequate efficiency in the surroundings for the regulation of the circadian rhythm.

Additionally, every one of us is aware that the daylighting has an important contribution to our health and well-being due to the improved quality of our environment. A pan-European (Velux 2015) survey determined that the Europeans living in dark buildings are more likely to report poor health compared to those who do not live in dark homes. One of the findings of the survey is that Europeans value daylight in the home. If they were to choose a new home, 47% would give the highest importance to the amount of daylight, 92% would give it above average importance, resulting in an indicator score of 6.1 out of 7. With greater age comes a greater appreciation of daylight in the home. Europeans also invest in improving daylight. More than one in four Europeans 27% have made changes within the last five years aimed at improving the amount of daylight in their home.

2.6 Population Groups and Priority Environments

National renovation strategies often define the priority built environments for renovation. Selection of the priority environment for renovation is often based on the cost-effective approach, which identifies the energy performance of the existing buildings and energy improvements. Selection explicitly on the **health status of a building** is almost never the primary criteria for decision making. Interestingly, the owners guiding factor for the renovation of an apartment building is first comfort and second energy efficiency.

Studies on **unhealthy buildings and the adverse health effects** (Sahlberg et al. 2013; Takigawa et al. 2012; Araki et al. 2010; Engvall et al. 2001; Scheel et al. 2001) revealed that the most problematic environments among public buildings are:

- health-care facilities,
- schools, and
- kindergartens.

Vulnerable population groups are always present in all built environments, also general ones. Because of the sensitivity of these groups and public health protection, all built environments should have the same priority.

Vulnerable population groups are: *"those that are particularly sensitive to risk factors and who possess multiple, cumulative risk factors. They present a subgroup of the population that is more likely to develop health problems as a*

*result of exposure to risk or to have worse outcomes from these health prob-
lems than the rest of the population"* (Stanhope and Lancaster 2015, p. 719).

According to WHO (2017d), the particularly vulnerable are:

- children,
- pregnant women,
- elderly people,
- malnourished people, and
- people who are ill or immunocompromised.

The numbers of these vulnerable populations are increasing, not only as the
proportion of the uninsured grows but as the population ages. The health domains
of vulnerable populations can be divided into 3 categories regarding (Aday 1994):

- physical
- psychological, and
- social.

According to the categories, specific needs are defined that has to be fulfilled in a
specific priority environment (Table 2.2).

Children are one example of a vulnerable population group. They are more
susceptible to environmental hazards than healthy adults are for several reasons
(ATSDR 2016; WHO 2017d):

- Children have disproportionately heavy exposures to environmental toxicants.
- In relation to body weight, children drink more water, eat more food, and
  breathe more air than adults. Children in the first 6 months of life drink seven
  times as much water per kg of body weight, and 1–5-year-old children eat 3–4
  times more food per kg than the average adult.
- The air intake of a resting infant is proportionally twice that of an adult. As a
  result, children will have substantially heavier exposures than adults to any
  toxicants that are present in water, food, or air.
- Two additional characteristics of children further magnify their exposures: their
  hand-to-mouth behaviour, and the fact that they live and play close to the
  ground.
- Children's metabolic pathways, especially in the first months after birth, are
  immature.
- Children's ability to metabolize, detoxify, and excrete many toxicants is different from that of adults. Commonly, however, they are less well able to deal
  with toxic chemicals and thus are more vulnerable to them.

Another vulnerable group is the **elderly**. Both internal and external factors can
contribute to the vulnerability of the elderly (Lachs and Pillemer 1995).

Table 2.2 Health domain, specific need, vulnerable population and priority environment (Aday 1994)

Health domain	Need	Vulnerable population	Priority environment
Physical	Physical	High-risk mothers and infants, the chronically ill and disabled, and persons living with HIV/ acquired immunodeficiency syndrome Chronic medical conditions include respiratory diseases, diabetes, hypertension, dyslipidaemia, and heart disease Elderly	Medical buildings (i.e. hospital, nursing home, rehabilitation) Residential buildings (i.e., apartment block, house, block of flats)
Psychological	Psychological	Populations with chronic mental conditions, such as schizophrenia, bipolar disorder, major depression, and attention-deficit/hyperactivity disorder Populations with a history of alcohol and/or substance abuse and those who are suicidal or prone to homelessness	Commercial buildings (i.e., shop, office, hotel, restaurant, gym) Educational buildings (school, museum, library) Governmental buildings (post office, parliament)
Social	Social	Populations of those living in abusive families, the homeless, immigrants, and refugees	Religious buildings (church, cathedral) Outdoor places (parks) Others

- **Internal risk factors include**: increasing age, female gender, medical comorbidities, substance abuse, mental illness, cognitive impairment, sensory impairment, impairment in activities of daily living (ADL), malnutrition.
- **External risk factors include**: lack of social network, dependence on a care provider, living alone, lack of community resources, inadequate housing, unsanitary living conditions, high-crime neighbourhood, adverse life events, poverty.

In the United States, 87% of those 65 years and older have one or more chronic conditions, and 67% of this population has two or more chronic illnesses (Partnership for Solutions 2002). Major chronic conditions affecting older people worldwide are cardiovascular disease, hypertension, stroke, diabetes, cancer, chronic obstructive pulmonary disease, musculoskeletal conditions, mental health condition, blindness and visual impairments (WHO 2002).

Globally, between 1970 and 2025, an increase in older persons of some 694 million or 223% is expected (WHO 2002). In Europe, the shift in the age pyramid is more dramatic: almost one third of people will be elderly in 2050. Due to dramatic demographic changes, the significant burden of dementia, chronically ill and immobile persons is expected. The **Survey of Health, Ageing and Retirement in Europe (SHARE)** showed that living conditions before and after retirement vary considerably across Europe and are not fully adjusted to the needs of the elderly (Börsch-Supan 2016). Therefore, the built environment must be adapted and designed for the future of society.

> **Each vulnerable group, as well as each individual in the group, has specific needs and requirements. If certain requirements and needs of users in a specific environment are not fulfilled, it can be severely debilitating or life-threatening.**

For example, a ward for severe **burn injuries** should have temperature controls that permit adjusting room air temperature up to 32 °C and relative air humidity up to 95% (ASHRAE Handbook 2007). The reason is that patients with large burn injuries have higher risks of hypermetabolism, hypothermia, higher evaporative water losses, progressive weight loss, increased susceptibility to infection, and poor wound healing (Corallo et al. 2007; Herndon and Tompkins 2004; Ramos et al. 2002; Herndon 1996, 1981; Kelemen 1996; Wallace et al. 1994; Caldwel et al. 1992; Carlson et al. 1992; Martin et al. 1992; Wilmore et al. 1975). To decrease energy demands, minimize metabolic expenditure and decrease the hypermetabolic response to thermal injury and evaporative water losses, room air temperature and relative air humidity should be maintained at 28–33 °C and 80%, respectively. In this way, optimal healing and comfort conditions are created (Dovjak 2012) and consequently mortality, morbidity, and hospitalization can be significantly decreased (Herndon 1996; Wilmore et al. 1975).

In current planning, it often happens that these needs tend to be underestimated. Current built environments are not meeting the needs of these vulnerable populations. The environment must be designed to take into account the rationales and requirements of a specific population group. The design of built environments following the concept of active **aging or age-friendly environment** is a good example.

> **An age-friendly environment** allows people to realize their potential for physical, social and mental well-being throughout the life course and to participate in society according to their needs, desires and capacities, while providing them with adequate protection, security and care when they require assistance (WHO 2002, p. 12).

A series of pan-European surveys, Velux (2017) determined that the link between adverse health effects and the indoor climate does not appear to be well known amongst Europeans, nor does the importance of correct behaviour.

Therefore, **health promotion with public awareness is a key to the successful prevention of adverse health effects**.

Public health is the science and art of preventing disease, prolonging life and promoting health through the organized efforts and informed choices of society, organizations, public and private, communities and individuals (Fink 2013, p. 2).

To summarize, various health outcomes are related to unhealthy built environments. SBS is one of the most researched health outcomes related to such environments. It is a consequence of exposure to numerous health risk factors and their parameters. The identification of health hazards and their parameters is the key step in the process of effective control and prevention. Therefore, on the basis of a comprehensive literature review, health risk factors and their parameters are systematically presented and classified in Chap. 3.

References

Aday, L. A. (1994). Health status of vulnerable populations, Who are the vulnerable? *Annual Review of Public Health, 15*, 487–509. Retrieved November 9, 2018, from http://www. annualreviews.org/doi/pdf/10.1146/annurev.pu.15.050194.002415. http://dx.doi.org/10.1146/ annurev.pu.15.050194.002415.

Araki, A., Kawai, T., Eitaki, Y., Kanazawa, A., Morimoto, K., Nakayama, K., et al. (2010). Relationship between selected indoor volatile organic compounds, so-called microbial VOC, and the prevalence of mucous membrane symptoms in single family homes. *Science of The Total Environment, 408*, 2208–2215. https://doi.org/10.1016/j.scitotenv.2010.02.012.

ASHRAE. (2013). *Standard 55-2013 Thermal environmental conditions for human occupancy.* Atlanta, GA: American Society of Heating, Refrigerating and Air-Conditioning Engineers Inc.

ASHRAE Handbook. (2007). *HVAC applications: Health care facilities. American Society of Heating.* (p. 1039) Atlanta, GA: Refrigerating and Air–Conditioning Engineers Inc.

ATSDR. (2016). *Agency for toxic substances disease registry principles of pediatric environmental health. What are factors affecting children's susceptibility to exposures?* Retrieved November 9, 2018, from https://www.atsdr.cdc.gov/csem/csem.asp?csem=27&po=6.

Barton, H., & Grant, M. (2006). A health map for the local human habitat. *The Journal for the Royal Society for the Promotion of Health, 126*(6), 252–253. https://doi.org/10.1177/ 1466424006070466.

Basagaña, X., Sartini, C., Barrera-Gómez, J., Dadvand, P., Cunillera, J., Ostro, B., et al. (2011). Heat waves and cause-specific mortality at all ages. *Epidemiology, 22*, 765–772. https://doi. org/10.1097/EDE.0b013e31823031c5.

Basner, M., Babisch, W., Davis, A., Brink, M., Clark, C., Janssen, S., et al. (2014). Auditory and non-auditory effects of noise on health. *Lancet, 383*(9925), 1325–1332.

Berson, D. M., Dunn, F. A., & Takao, M. (2002). Phototransduction by Retinal Ganglion cells that set the circadian clock. *Science, 295*(5557), 1070–1073. https://doi.org/10.1126/science. 1067262.

Bourbeau, J., Brisson, C., & Allaire, S. (1997). Prevalence of the sick building syndrome symptoms in office workers before and six months and three years after being exposed to a building with an improved ventilation system. *Occupational and Environmental Medicine, 54,* 49–53. https://doi.org/10.1136/oem.54.1.49.

Börsch-Supan, A. (2016). *Survey of Health, Ageing and Retirement in Europe (SHARE) Wave 5. Release version: 5.0.0.* SHARE-ERIC. Data set.

Bossel, H. (1999). *Indicators for sustainable development: Theory, method, applications, a report to the Balaton group.* International Institute for Sustainable Development, Canada, p. 138.

BPIE. (2014). *Buildings Performance Institute Europe. Alleviating fuel poverty in the EU investing in home renovation, a sustainable and inclusive solution.* Retrieved November 9, 2018, from http://bpie.eu/wp-content/uploads/2015/10/Alleviating-fuel-poverty.pdf.

Brandis, K. (2013). *Fluid Physiology. Anaesthesia Education Website.* Retrieved November 9, 2018, from http://www.anaesthesiaMCQ.com.

Braubach, M., Jackobs. D. E., & Ormandy, D. (2011) *Environmental burden of disease associated with inadequate housing.* Retrieved October 10, 2018, from http://www.euro.who.int/__data/assets/pdf_file/0003/142077/e95004.pdf.

Bresjanac, M., & Rupnik, M. (1999). *Patofiziologija s temelji fiziologije.* Ljubljana: Inštitut za patološko fiziologijo.

Burge, P. S. (2004). Sick building syndrome. *Occupational and Environmental Medicine, 61,* 185–190. https://doi.org/10.1136/oem.2003.008813.

Burge, S., Hedge, A., Wilson, S., Bass, J. H., & Robertson, A. (1987). Sick building syndrome: A study of 4373 office workers. *Annals of Occupational Hygiene, 31,* 493–504.

Caldwel, F. T., Wallace, B. H., Cone, J. B., & Manuel, L. (1992). Control of the hypermetabolic response to burn injury using environmental factors. *Annals of Surgery, 215*(5), 485–491. https://doi.org/10.1097/00000658-199205000-00011.

Cannon, W. B. (1926). *Physiological regulation of normal states: Some Tentative Postulates Concerning Biological Homeostatics.* Paris: Éditions Médicales.

Carlson, D. E., Cioffi, W. G., & Mason, A. D. (1992). Resting energy expenditure in patients with thermal injuries. *Surgery, Gynecology and Obstetrics, 174,* 270–276.

Clark, L. A., & Watson, D. J. (1988). Mood and the mundane: Relations between daily life events and self-reported mood. *Personality and Social Psychology, 54*(2), 296–308. https://doi.org/10.1037/0022-3514.54.2.296.

Corallo, J., King, B., Pizano, L., Namias, N., & Schulman, C. (2007). Core warming of a burn patient during excision to prevent hypothermia. *Burns, 34*(3), 418–420. https://doi.org/10.1016/j.burns.2007.08.012.

CPR 305/2011/EU Regulation (EU) No 305/2011 of the European Parliament and of the Council of 9 March 2011laying down harmonised conditions for the marketing of construction products an repealing Council Directive 89/106/EEC. Retrieved October 10, 2018, from http://eurlex.europa.eu/legalcontent/SL/TXT/?uri=CELEX%3A32011R0305.

Crystal Palace Building, London, United Kingdom. (2008). Retrieved November 9, 2018, from https://www.britannica.com/topic/Crystal-Palace-building-London.

Dahlgren, G., & Whitehead, M. (1991). *Policies and strategies to promote social equity in health.* Stockholm, Sweden: Institute for Future Studies.

Directive 2001/42/EC of the European Parliament and of the Council of 27 June 2001 on the assessment of the effects of certain plans and programmes on the environment (SEA Directive).

Directive 2011/92/EU of the European Parliament and of the Council of 13 December 2011 on the assessment of the effects of certain public and private projects on the environment.

Ding, G. K. C. (2008). Sustainable construction—The role of environmental assessment tools. *Journal of Environmental Management, 86,* 451–464. https://doi.org/10.1016/j.jenvman.2006.12.025.

Dovjak, M. (2012). *Individualisation of personal space in hospital environment: Doctoral dissertation.* Nova Gorica: University of Nova Gorica.

Dovjak, M., Kukec, A., Kristl, Ž., Košir, M., Bilban, M., Shukuya, M., et al. (2013). Integral control of health hazards in hospital environment. *Indoor and Built Environment, 22*(5), 776–795. https://doi.org/10.1177/1420326X1245986.

Dovjak, M., Krainer, A., & Shukuya, M. (2014). Individualisation of personal space in hospital environment. *International Journal of Exergy, 14*(2), 125–155. https://doi.org/10.1504/IJEX. 2014.060279.

EC. (1992). Towards Sustainability: A European Community Programme of Policy and Action in Relation to the Environment and Sustainable Development. Volume 2. Executive Summary, Commission of the European Communities, Brussels, p. 93.

EC. (2007). *Health & Consumer Protection Directorate-General, Opinion on risk assessment on indoor air quality*. Retrieved October 10, 2018, from http://ec.europa.eu/health/ph_risk/ committees/04_scher/docs/scher_o_055.pdf.

ECA. (1989). *Indoor air quality & its impact on man. COST Project 613, Environment and Quality of Life Report No. 4, Sick Building Syndrome, A Practical Guide. Commission of the European Communities, Directorate General for Science, Research and Development, Joint Research Centre—Institute for the Environment*. Commission of the European Communities, Luxembourg. Retrieved October 10, 2018, from http://www.buildingecology.com/ publications/ECA_Report4.pdf.

Engvall, K., Norrby, C., & Norbäck, D. (2001). Sick building syndrome in relation to building dampness in multi-family residential buildings in Stockholm. *International Archives of Occupational and Environmental Health, 74,* 270–278.

EPA. (1991). I*ndoor Air Facts No. 4 (revised), Sick Building Syndrome. United States Environmental Air and Radiation*. Retrieved October 10, 2018, from https://www.epa.gov/ sites/production/files/201408/documents/sick_building_factsheet.pdf.

EPA. (2009). *Green Building Basic Information*. Retrieved October 10, 2018, from http://www. epa.gov/greenbuilding/pubs/about.html.

EPA. (2017). *Indoor Air Quality (IAQ). The Inside Story: A Guide to Indoor Air Quality*. Retrieved October 10, 2018, from https://www.epa.gov/indoor-air-quality-iaq/inside-story-guide-indoor-air-quality.

Eržen, I., Gajšek, P., Hlastan Ribič, C., Kukec, A., Poljšak, B., & Zaletel Kragelj, L. (2010). *Zdravje in okolje: Izbrana poglavja*. Medicinska fakulteta, Maribor: Univerza v Mariboru.

Espiritu, R. C., Kripke, D. F., Ancoli-Israel, S., Mowen, M. A., Mason, W. J., Fell, R. L., et al. (1994). Low illumination experienced by San Diego adults: Association with atypical depressive symptoms. *Biological Psychiatry, 35*(6), 403–407. https://doi.org/10.1016/0006-3223(94)90007-8.

Evans, R. G., & Stoddart, G. L. (1990). Producing health, consuming health care. *Social Science and Medicine, 31,* 1347–1363. https://doi.org/10.1016/0277-9536(90)90074-3.

Fanger, P. O. (1970). *Thermal comfort*. Copenhagen: Danish Technical Press.

Fink, A. G. (2013). *Evidence-based public health practice*. California: University of California, The Langley Research Institute, SAGE Publications Inc.

Fisk, W. J., Eliseeva, E. A., & Mendell, M. J. (2010). Association of residential dampness and mold with respiratory tract infections and bronchitis: A meta-analysis. *Environmental Health, 15*(9), 72–84. https://doi.org/10.1186/1476-069X-9-72.

Fitwel (n.d.). *The Cost-Effective, High-Impact Building Certification*. Retrieved October 10, 2018, from https://fitwel.org.

Forsberg, A., & von Malmborg, F. (2004). Tools for environmental assessment of the built environment. *Building and Environment, 39,* 223–228. https://doi.org/10.1016/j.buildenv. 2003.09.004.

Gagge, A. P., Stolwijk, J., & Hardy, J. (1967). Comfort and thermal sensations and associated physiological responses at various ambient temperatures. *Environmental Research, 1*(1), 1–20. https://doi.org/10.1016/0013-9351(67)90002-3.

Geng, Y., Ji, W., Lin, B., & Zhu, Y. (2017). The impact of thermal environment on occupant IEQ perception and productivity. *Building and Environment, 121,* 158–167. https://doi.org/10.1016/j.buildenv.2017.05.022.

Healy, J. D. (2003). Excess winter mortality in Europe: A cross country analysis identifying key risk factors. *Journal of Epidemiology and Community Health, 57,* 784–789. Retrieved October 10, 2018, from http://jech.bmj.com/content/jech/57/10/784.full.pdf. http://dx.doi.org/10.1136/jech.57.10.784.

Heerwagen, J. H. (1986). *The role of nature in the view from the window.* In S. Zdepski, & R. McCluney (Eds.) (1986) *International Daylighting Conference Proceedings II,* November 4–7, 1986. International Daylighting Organizing Committee, Long Beach, CA, pp. 430–437.

Herndon, D. N. (1981). Mediators of metabolism. *Journal of Trauma, 21,* 701–705. https://doi.org/10.1097/00005373-198108001-00024.

Herndon, D. N. (1996). *Total burn care* (1st ed.). London: Sunders.

Herndon, D. N., & Tompkins, R. G. (2004). Support of the metabolic response to burn injury. *Lancet, 363*(9424), 1895–1902.

Ho, D. C. W., Leung, H. F., Wong, S. K., Cheung, A. K. C., Lau, S. S. Y., Wong, W. S., et al. (2004). Assessing the health and hygiene performance of apartment buildings. *Facilities, 22*(3/4), 58–69. https://doi.org/10.1108/02632770410527789.

Hwang, R. L., Lin, T. P., Cheng, M. J., & Chien, J. H. (2007). Patient thermal comfort requirement for hospital environments in Taiwan. *Building and Environment, 42*(8), 2980–2987. https://doi.org/10.1016/j.buildenv.2006.07.035.

Institute of Medicine. (1997). *Improving health in the community: A role for performance monitoring.* Institute of Medicine (US) Committee on Using Performance Monitoring to Improve Community Health.

IPHA. (2018). *International Passive House Association.* Passive House certification criteria. Retrieved July 9, 2018, from https://www.passivehouse-international.org/index.php?page_id=150.

ISO 7730:2005 Ergonomics of the thermal environment -Analytical determination and interpretation of thermal comfort using calculation of the PMV and PPD indices and local thermal comfort criteria.

Jantunen, M., Oliveira Fernandes, E., Carrer, P., & Kephalopoulos, S. (2011). *Promoting actions for healthy indoor air (IAIAQ).* Luxembourg: European Commission Directorate General for Health and Consumers. Retrieved October 10, 2018, from https://ec.europa.eu/health//sites/health/files/healthy_environments/docs/env_iaiaq.pdf.

Jeffery, R. D. (2013). Adverse health effects of industrial wind turbines. *Can Fam Physician, 59*(5), 473–475.

Jenkins, D., & Newborough, M. (2007). An approach for estimating the carbon emissions associated with office lighting with a daylight contribution. *Applied Energy, 84*(6), 608–622. https://doi.org/10.1016/j.apenergy.2007.02.002.

Karjalainen, S. (2007). Gender differences in thermal comfort and use of thermostats in everyday thermal environments. *Building and Environment, 42*(4), 1594–1603. https://doi.org/10.1016/j.buildenv.2006.01.009.

Kelemen, J. J., Cioffi, W. G., Mason, A. D., Mozingo, D. W., McManus, W. F., & Pruitt, B. A. (1996). Effect of ambient temperature on metabolic rate after thermal injury. *Annals of Surgery, 223,* 406–412. https://doi.org/10.1097/00000658-199604000-00009.

Kim, J. T. (2012). Sustainable and healthy buildings. *Energ Buildings, 46,* 1–2. https://doi.org/10.1016/j.enbuild.2011.10.032.

Kingsley, S. L., Eliot, M. N., Gold, J., Vanderslice, R. R., & Wellenius, G. A. (2016). Current and projected heat-related morbidity and mortality in Rhode Island. *Environmental Health Perspectives, 124,* 460–467. https://doi.org/10.1289/ehp.1408826.

Klepeis, N. E., Nelson, W. C., Ott, W. R., Robinson, J. P., Tsang, A. M., Switzer, P., et al. (2001). The national human activity pattern survey (NHAPS): A resource for assessing exposure to environmental pollutants. *Journal of Exposure Analysis and Environmental Epidemiology, 11*(3), 231–252. https://doi.org/10.1038/sj.jea.7500165.

Kukec, A., Krainer, A., & Dovjak, M. (2015). Possible adverse effects of building dampness on occupants' health. *Gradbeni vestnik, 64*, 36–46.

Lachs, M. S., & Pillemer, K. (1995). Abuse and neglect of elderly persons. *N Engl J Med, 332*, 437–443. https://doi.org/10.1056/NEJM199502163320706.

Lan, L., Wargocki, P., & Lian, Z. (2012). *Optimal thermal environment improves performance of office work*. REHVA. Retrieved October 10, 2018, from http://www.rehva.eu/index.php?id=151.

Last, J. M. *A Dictionary of epidemiology*. (4th edn) (2001) New York Oxford: University Press.

Larson, L. R., Green, T. G., & Cordell, H. K. (2011). Children's time outdoors: Results and implications of the National Kids Survey. *Journal of Park and Recreation Administration, 29*, 1–20.

Lavin, T., Higgins, C., Metcalfe, O., & Jordan, A. (2006). *Health Impacts of the Built Environment, a review*. Institute of Public Health in Ireland. Retrieved October 10, 2018, from http://www.publichealth.ie/files/file/Health_Impacts_of_the_Built_Environment_A_Review.pdf.

Leech, J. A., Wilby, K., McMullen, E., & Laporte, K. (1996). The Canadian Human Activity Pattern Survey: A report of methods and population surveyed. *Chronic Dis Can, 17*(3–4), 118–123.

Living Building Challenge. (2017). *International living future*. Retrieved November 4, 2018, from http://living-future.org/lbc.

Loftness, V., Hakkinen, B., Adan, O., & Nevalainen Adan, O. (2007). Elements that contribute to healthy building design. *Environmental Health Perspectives, 115*(6), 965–970. Retrieved October 10, 2018, from https://www.ncbi.nlm.nih.gov/pmc/articles/PMC1892106/. http://dx.doi.org/10.1289/ehp.8988.

Magnusson, A. (2000). An overview of epidemiological studies on seasonal affective disorder. *Acta Psychiatrica Scandinavica, 101*(3), 176–184. https://doi.org/10.1034/j.1600-0447.2000.101003176.x.

Manfred, A. M. N., Elizalde, A., & Hopenhayn, M. (1989). *Human scale development: Conception, Application and Further Reflections*. Apex. Press Chpt. 2. Development and Human Needs, New York, p. 18.

Mao, P., Qi, J., Tan, Y., & Lia, J. (2017). An examination of factors affecting healthy building: An empirical study in east China. *The Journal of Cleaner Production, 162*, 1266–1274.

Martin, C. J., Ferguson, J. C., & Rayner, C. (1992). Environmental conditions for treatment of burned patients by the exposure method. *Burns, 18*, 273–282. https://doi.org/10.1016/0305-4179(92)90147-M.

Markelj, J., Kitek Kuzman, M., Grošelj, P., & Zbašnik-Senegačnik, M. (2014). A simplified method for evaluating building sustainability in the early design phase for architects. *Sustainability, 6*(12), 775–8795. https://doi.org/10.3390/su6128775.

Maslow, A. H. (1943). A theory of human motivation. *Psychological Review, 50*(4), 370–396. https://doi.org/10.1037/h0054346.

Marmot Review Team. (2011). *The Health Impacts of Cold Homes and Fuel Poverty*. Retrieved October 10, 2018, from https://www.foe.co.uk/sites/default/files/downloads/cold_homes_health.pdf.

Medical dictionary Health. (2017). Retrieved October 10, 2018, from http://medical-dictionary.thefreedictionary.com/health.

Melikov, A. K., Cermak, R., & Majer, M. (2002). Personalized ventilation: Evaluation of different air terminal devices. *Energy and Buildings, 34*(8), 829–836. https://doi.org/10.1016/S0378-7788(02)00102-0.

Mersch, P. P., Middendorp, H. M., Bouhuys, A. L., Beersma, D. G., & van den Hoofdakker, R. H. (1999). Seasonal affective disorder and latitude: A review of the literature. *Journal of Affective Disorders, 53*(1), 35–48. https://doi.org/10.1016/S0165-0327(98)00097-4.

Milan. (2012). *Milan overview, Insight Guides website*. London, England, U.K.: Apa Publications UK, 2012. Retrieved February 6, 2018, fromhttps://www.insightguides.com/destinations/europe/italy/the-northwest/milan.

Mohtashami, N., Mahdavinejad, M., & Bemanian, M. (2016). Contribution of City prosperity to decisions on healthy building design: A case study of Tehran. *Frontiers of Architectural Research, 5*(3), 319–331. https://doi.org/10.1016/j.foar.2016.06.001.

Mudarri, D., & Fisk, W. J. (2007). Public health and economic impact of dampness and mold. *Indoor Air, 17*(3), 226–235. https://doi.org/10.1111/j.1600-0668.2007.00474.x.

Musek, J., & Pečjak, V. (2001). *Psychology*. Ljubljana: Educy.

Naci, H., & Ioannidis, J. P. (2015). Evaluation of Wellness Determinants and Interventions by Citizen Scientists. *JAMA, 314*(2), 121–122. https://doi.org/10.1001/jama.2015.6160.

Novick, R. (1999). *Overview of the environment and health in Europe in the 1990s*. World Health Organisation, Geneva. Retrieved February 6, 2018 from http://www.euro.who.int/document/e66792.pdf.

Oxford Dictionaries. (2017). Retrieved October 10, 2018, from https://en.oxforddictionaries.com/definition/comfort.

Parsons, K. C. (2002). The effects of gender, acclimation state, the opportunity to adjust clothing and physical disability on requirements for thermal comfort. *Energ Buildings, 34*(6), 593–599. https://doi.org/10.1016/S0378-7788(02)00009-9.

Parsons, K. (2014). *Human thermal environments* (3rd ed.). Boca Raton, FL: CRC Press.

Partnership for Solutions. (2002). *Chronic conditions: Making the case for ongoing care*. Johns Hopkins University. Retrieved February 8, 2018 from http://www.kff.org/uninsured/upload/covering-the-uninsured-growing-need-strained-resources-fact-sheet.pdf.

Pirastu, R., Bellu, C., Greco, P., Pelosi, U., Pistelli, R., Accetta, G., et al. (2009). Indoor exposure to environmental tobacco smoke and dampness: Respiratory symptoms in Sardinian children— DRIAS study. *Environmental Research, 109,* 59–65. https://doi.org/10.1016/j.envres.2008.09.002.

Pirhonen, I., Nevalainen, A., Husman, T., & Pekkanen, J. (1996). Home dampness, moulds and their influence on respiratory infections and symptoms in adults in Finland. *European Respiratory Journal, 9,* 2618–2622. https://doi.org/10.1183/09031936.96.09122618.

Potrč, T., Kunič, R., Legat, A., & Dovjak, M. (2017). Health aspects in building certification systems. In Proceedings of the 1st International Conference CoMS_2017, 19-21 April 2017, Zadar, Croatia, pp. 878–889.

Prek, M., & Butala, V. (2012). An enhanced thermal comfort model based on the exergy analysis approach. *The International Journal of Exergy, 10*(2), 190–208. https://doi.org/10.1504/IJEX.2012.045865.

Public health England. (2016). *Active aging*. Retrieved October 10, 2018, from https://www.google.si/?gws_rd=cr&ei=Ny93WaCPKMbPwAKIIIuwDw#q=active+aging+and+the+built+environment.

Ramos, G. E., Resta, M., Patiño, O., Bolgiani, A. N., Prezzavento, G., Grillo, R., et al. (2002). Peri –operative hypothermia in burn patients subjected to non –extensive surgical procedures. *Annals of Burns and Fire Disasters, 15*(3), 1–6.

Rasmussen, B. (2010). *Sound classification schemes in EU-Quality classes intended for renovated building*. Retrieved October 11, 2018, from http://vbn.aau.dk/files/43741580/SoundClassesEuropeRenovatedHousing_TU0701_UniversityMalta_May2010BiR.pdf.

Redlich, C. A., Sparer, J., & Cullen, M. R. (1997). Sick-building syndrome. *The Lancet, 349,* 1013–1016. https://doi.org/10.1016/S0140-6736(96)07220-0.

Ribble Cycles survey. (2017). Retrieved October 10, 2018, from https://www.ribblecycles.co.uk/bikes/.

Rio Declaration. (1992). *Rio Declaration on Environment and Development*. The United Nations Conference on Environment and Development, Rio de Janeiro from 3 to 14 June 1992.

Robbins, C. L. (1986). *Daylighting: Design and analysis* (pp. 4–13). New York: Van Nostrand Reinhold Company.

Robinson, J. P., & Thomas, J. (1991). *Time spent in activities, locations, and microenvironments: A California- national comparison*. United States Environmental Protection Agency, Final EPA Report, Washington, DC.

Rosen, L., Targum, S., Terman, M., Bryant. M. J., Hoffman, H., Kasper, S. F., et al. (1990). Prevalence of seasonal affective disorder at four latitudes. *Psychiatry Research, 31*(2), 131–144. http://dx.doi.org/10.1016/0165-1781(90)90116-M http://dx.doi.org/10.1016/0165-1781 (90)90116-M.

Roecklein, K. A., & Rohan, K. J. (2005). Seasonal affective disorder. *An Overview and Update. Psychiatry (Edgmont), 2*(1), 20–26.

Ryff, C., & Keyes, C. (1995). The structure of psychological well-being revisited. *Journal of Personality and Social Psychology, 69,* 719–727. https://doi.org/10.1037/0022-3514.69.4.719.

Sahlberg, B., Gunnbjörnsdottir, M., Soon, A., Jogi, R., Gislason, T., Wieslander, G., et al. (2013). Airborne molds and bacteria, microbial volatile organic compounds (MVOC), plasticizers and formaldehyde in dwellings in three North European cities in relation to sick building syndrome (SBS). *Science of the Total Environment, 444,* 433–440. https://doi.org/10.1016/j.scitotenv. 2012.10.114.

Scheel, C. M., Rosing, W. C., & Farone, A. L. (2001). Possible sources of sick building syndrome in a tennessee middle school. *Archives of Environmental Health, 56,* 413–417.

Schellen, L., van Marken Lichtenbelt, W. D., Loomans, M. G., Toftum, J., & de Wit, M. H. (2010). Differences between young adults and elderly in thermal comfort, productivity, and thermal physiology in response to a moderate temperature drift and a steady-state condition. *Indoor Air, 20*(4), 273–283. https://doi.org/10.1111/j.1600-0668.2010.00657.x.

Schellen, L., Loomans, M. G., de Wit, M. H., Olesen, B. W., & van Marken Lichtenbelt, W. D. (2012). The influence of local effects on thermal sensation under non-uniform environmental conditions-gender differences in thermophysiology, thermal comfort and productivity during convective and radiant cooling. *Physiology & Behavior, 107*(2), 252–261. https://doi.org/10. 1016/j.physbeh.2012.07.008.

Schweiker, M., Carlucci, S., Andersen, R., Dong, B., & O'Brien, W. (2018). *Occupancy and occupants' actions in exploring occupant behaviour in buildings: Methods and challenges.* Cham: Springer.

Shukuya, M. (2013). *Exergy.* Theory and Applications in the Built Environment. Springer, Springer London Heidelberg New York Dordrecht.

Silverman, W. A., Fertig, J. W., & Berger, A. P. (1958). The influence of thermal environment on survival of newly born premature infant. *Pediatrics, 22,* 876–886.

Simone, A., Kolarik, J., Iwamatsu, T., Asada, H., Dovjak, M., Schellen, L., et al. (2011). A relation between calculated human body exergy consumption rate and subjectively assessed thermal sensation. *Energy Build, 43*(1), 1–9. https://doi.org/10.1016/j.enbuild.2010.08.007.

Skoog, J., Fransson, N., & Jagemar, L. (2005). Thermal environment in Swedish hospitals summer and winter measurements. *Energy and Buildings, 37*(8), 872–877. https://doi.org/10.1016/j. enbuild.2004.11.003.

Smith. (1993). Fuel combustion, air pollution exposure, and health: The situation in developing countries. *Annual Review of Environment, 18*: 529–566.

Smajlović, K., Dovjak, M., & Kukec, A. (2019). *Prevalence of sick building syndrome in hospitals in relation to environmental factors: Literature review.* Slovenian Nursing Review (in press).

Stanhope, M., & Lancaster, J. (2015). *Public Health Nursing—E-Book: Population-Centered Health Care in the Community 9th Edition.* Mosby.

Stevens and Hall. (1993). Environmental health. In J. Swanson & M. Albracht (Eds.), *Community health nursing.* Philadelphia: WB Saunders.

SustainableBuild. (2017). *What is Eco Friendly Construction?* Retrieved October 10, 2018, from http://www.sustainablebuild.co.uk/ecofriendlyconstruction.html.

Takigawa, T., Saijo, Y., Morimoto, K., Nakayama, K., Shibata, E., Tanaka, M., et al. (2012). A longitudinal study of aldehydes and volatile organic compounds associated with subjective symptoms related to sick building syndrome in new dwellings in Japan. *Science of the Total Environment, 417–418,* 61–67. https://doi.org/10.1016/j.scitotenv.2011.12.060.

The Economist. (2004). *The rise of the green building.* Retrieved October 10, 2018, from http:// www.economist.com/node/3422965.

The Guardian. (2016). *Children spend only half as much time playing outside as their parents did*. Retrieved October 10, 2018, from https://www.theguardian.com/environment/2016/jul/27/children-spend-only-half-the-time-playing-outside-as-their-parents-did.

Topp, C. W., Østergaard, S. D., Søndergaard, S., & Bech, P. (2015). The WHO-5 Well-Being Index: A systematic review of the literature. *Psychother Psychosom, 84*(3), 167–176. https://doi.org/10.1159/000376585.

Tov, W., & Diener. (2013). *Subjective Well-Being. Research Collection School of Social Sciences*. Paper 1395. Retrieved October 10, 2018, from http://ink.library.smu.edu.sg/soss_research/1395.

Turner, S. (2016). *Healthy buildings international*. Healthy Buildings Core Purpose. Inc. and Healthy Building Solutions, LLC. Retrieved November 2, 2018, from http://healthybuildings.com/.

Velux. (2015). *The Healthy Homes Barometer 2015*. Retrieved October 10, 2018, from http://www.velux.com/article/2016/energy-renovation-resonates-with-european-home-owners.

Velux. (2017). *Healthy Homes Barometer 2017 Buildings and Their Impact on the Health of Europeans*. Retrieved October 10, 2018, from http://velcdn.azureedge.net/~/media/com/health/healthy-home-barometer/507505-01%20barometer_2017.pdf.

Wallace, B. H., Caldwell, F. T., & Cone, J. B. (1994). The interrelationships between wound management, thermal stress, energy metabolism, and temperature profiles of patients with burns. *The Journal of Burn Care & Rehabilitation, 15*(6), 499–508.

WCED. (1987). Report of the World Commission on Environment and Development. World Commission on Environment and Development. Brundtland Commission.

WELL. (2016). *WELL Greenbuild*. Retrieved October 4, 2018, from https://www.wellcertified.com/.

WGBC. (2014). *World Green Building Council—Health, Wellbeing and Productivity in Offices*. Retrieved April 11, 2018, from http://www.worldgbc.org/files/9714/3401/7431/WorldGBC_Health_Wellbeing__Productivity_Full_Report_.

WHECA. (2000). *Warm Homes and Energy Conservation Act 2000*.

WHO. (1946). *Preamble to the Constitution of WHO as adopted by the International Health Conference*. Retrieved October 10, 2018, from https://www.ncbi.nlm.nih.gov/pmc/articles/PMC2567705/pdf/12571729.pdf.

WHO. (1983). Indoor air pollutants: Exposure and health effects, EURO Reports and Studies No. 78, World Health Organisation, Regional Office for Europe, Copenhagen.

WHO. (1986). A discussion document on the concept and principles of health promotion. *Health Promotion, 1*(1), 73–78.

WHO. (1989). *Environment and health: A European charter and commentary*. Copenhagen: WHO.

WHO. (1992). Our planet, our health Report of the WHO Commission on Health and Environment. World Health Organisation. Geneva. Retrieved October 10, 2018, from http://apps.who.int/iris/bitstream/10665/37933/1/9241561483.pdf.

WHO. (1998). *Health Promotion Glossary. World Health Organisation, Geneva*. Retrieved October 10, 2018, from http://www.who.int/healthpromotion/about/HPR%20Glossary%201998.pdf.

WHO. (2001). *ICF International Classification of Functioning, Disability and Health (ICF)*. Retrieved October 10, 2018, from http://www.who.int/classifications/icf/en/.

WHO. (2002). *Active aging*. Retrieved October 10, 2018, from http://apps.who.int/iris/bitstream/10665/67215/1/WHO_NMH_NPH_02.8.pdf.

WHO. (2005). *Constitution of the WHO: Principles*. Retrieved October 10, 2018, from http://www.who.int/about/mission/en/.

WHO. (2009a). *Dampness and mould*. Retrieved October 10, 2018, from http://www.euro.who.int/__data/assets/pdf_file/0017/43325/E92645.pdf.

WHO. (2009b). *Night noise guidelines for Europe*. Retrieved October 10, 2018, from http://www.euro.who.int/__data/assets/pdf_file/0017/43316/E92845.pdf.

WHO. (2010). *WHO Guidelines for Indoor Air Quality*. Retrieved October 10, 2018, from http://www.euro.who.int/__data/assets/pdf_file/0009/128169/e94535.pdf.

WHO. (2011). *Burden of disease from environmental noise. Quantification of healthy life years lost in Europe*. Retrieved October 10, 2018, from http://www.euro.who.int/__data/assets/pdf_file/0008/136466/e94888.pdf.

WHO. (2016). *Household air pollution and health*. Retrieved October 10, 2018, from http://www.who.int/mediacentre/factsheets/fs292/en/.

WHO. (2017a). *Health Impact Assessment (HIA)*. Retrieved October 10, 2018, from http://www.who.int/hia/evidence/doh/en/.

WHO. (2017b). *WHOQOL: Measuring Quality of Life*. Retrieved October 10, 2018, from http://www.who.int/healthinfo/survey/whoqol-qualityoflife/en/.

WHO. (2017c). *Global Health Observatory (GHO) data*. Retrieved October 10, 2018, from http://www.who.int/gho/en/.

WHO. (2017d). *Environmental health in emergencies*. Vulnerable groups. Retrieved October 10, 2018, from http://www.who.int/environmental_health_emergencies/vulnerable_groups/en/.

Wilmore, D. W., Mason, A. D., Johnson, D. W., & Pruitt, B. A. (1975). Effect of ambient temperature on heat production and heat loss in burn patients. *Journal of Applied Physiology, 38*(4), 593–597. https://doi.org/10.1152/jappl.1975.38.4.593.

Woods, J., Drewry, G., & Morey, P. (1987). Office worker perceptions of indoor air quality effects on discomfort and performance. In *Proceedings of the 4th international Conference on Indoor Air and Climate. In 4th international Conference on Indoor Air and Climate*. Berlin, pp. 464–408.

Yassi, A., Kjellstrom, T., deKok, T., & Guidotti, T. (2001). *Basic environmental health*. New York: Oxford University Press.

Chapter 3
Identification of Health Risk Factors and Their Parameters

Abstract This chapter highlights the importance of identifying health risk factors and their parameters for healthier built environments. In Sect. 3.1, epidemiological terms such as "determinants of health", "health risk" and "health hazards", are introduced. In Sect. 3.2, health risk factors and their main parameters in built environments are further identified and classified into six groups: biological, chemical, physical, psychosocial, personal, and others. Detailed definition of health risk factors and their main parameters, followed by the results of epidemiological studies proving the association between potential health outcomes and health risk factors, are described in Sects. 3.3, 3.4, 3.5, 3.6 and 3.7. Identified and classified health risk factors and their parameters are the basis for the identification of single and multi-group interactions among them, described in Chap. 4.

3.1 Determinants of Health, Health Risk, and Health Hazard Factors

Whether people are healthy or not is determined by their circumstances and environment. WHO defines health risk factors from built environments, genetics, income and education levels, and relationships with friends and family. All these factors have considerable impacts on health, while other more commonly considered factors, such as access and use of health care services, often have less of an impact (WHO 2017a).

The determinants of built environments include:

- **Physical environment**,
- **Social and economic environment**, and
- **Person's individual characteristics and behaviours**.

Individuals often cannot control many of the **determinants of health** in built environments (Table 3.1).

"**Risk**" and "**hazard**" are terms commonly used to describe aspects of the potential harm to health. The terms "health risk" and "health hazard" are often not

© The Author(s) 2019
M. Dovjak and A. Kukec, *Creating Healthy and Sustainable Buildings*, https://doi.org/10.1007/978-3-030-19412-3_3

Table 3.1 Determinants of health in built environments (WHO 2017a)

Determinants of health	Link to health
Physical environment	Safe water and clean air, healthy workplaces, safe houses, communities and roads all contribute to good health
Income and social status	Higher income and social status are linked to better health. The greater the gap between the richest and poorest people, the greater the differences in health
Education	Low education levels are linked to poor health, more stress, and lower self-confidence
Employment and working conditions	People with employment are healthier, particularly those who have more control over their working conditions
Social support networks	Greater support from families, friends and communities is linked to better health
Personal behaviour and coping skills	Eating habits, level of physical activity, smoking, drinking, and how we deal with life's stresses and challenges all affect health
Culture	Customs, traditions, and the beliefs of the family and community all affect health
Genetics	Inheritance plays a part in determining lifespan, healthiness, and the likelihood of developing certain illnesses
Gender	Men and women suffer from different types of diseases at different ages
Health services	Access to and use of services that prevent and treat disease influence health

properly used. The term "**risk**" is the "likelihood that a person may be harmed or suffers adverse health effects if exposed to a **hazard**" (HSA 2017).

The level of risk is often categorized according to the potential harm or adverse health effect that the **hazard** may cause, how many times a person is exposed, and the number of persons exposed (HSA 2017). **Health hazards frequently occur in all built environments**. They may be in the form of chemical hazards (e.g., chlorine or a pesticide), biological hazards (e.g., fungi in damp buildings), physical hazards (e.g., excessive noise, coldness, over-heating or radiation), ergonomic hazards (e.g., unhealthy body positions and repetitive strain) and psychological hazards (e.g., anxiety) (Safeopedia 2017).

BOX 3.1 Health risk

The term "health risk" is defined as something that could cause harm to people's health (Collins 2017a, b). The Environmental Protection Agency (EPA 2016) considers risk to be: "The chance of harmful effects to human health or to ecological systems resulting from exposure to an environmental stressor". Therefore, **a human health risk** is described as: "The likelihood that a given exposure or series of exposures may have damaged or will damage the health of individuals" (EPA 2016).

BOX 3.2 Health hazard

A health hazard is defined as something that is dangerous to health. The most common definition of a health hazard is: "a potential source of harm or adverse health effect on a person(s)". For example, a place is structurally unsafe (Collins 2017b; HSA 2017).

For example, the leading **global risks for mortality** in the world are high blood pressure (responsible for 13% of deaths globally), tobacco use (9%), high blood glucose (6%), physical inactivity (6%), and overweight and obesity (5%) (WHO 2009a). As a country develops, the types of diseases that affect a population shift from primarily infectious illnesses, such as diarrhoea and pneumonia, to primarily noncommunicable illnesses, such as cardiovascular disease and cancers (WHO 2009a). Many diseases are caused by multiple risk factors, and individual risk factors may interact in their impact on the **overall risk of disease**. As a result, attributable fractions of deaths and burden for individual risk factors usually overlap and often add up to more than 100% (WHO 2009a). A prime example of this is that two risk factors—smoking and radon—cause lung cancer. Exposure to radon is the second leading cause of lung cancer (EPA 2017a). The risk is significantly higher for smokers than for non-smokers. Globally, more than 85% of radon-induced lung cancer deaths are among smokers. The optimal strategy for the elimination of the public health burden of radon includes building design strategies with remediation, residential radon testing as well as smoking prevention (Lantz et al. 2013).

Some **risk factors** can be changed, such as unhealthy lifestyle habits and environments. Other risk factors, such as age, family history and genetics, race and ethnicity, and sex, cannot be changed. Healthy lifestyle changes as well as a healthy environment can decrease your risk for developing some diseases (NIH 2017). It is clear that many **environmental factors** can affect health. For example, some of the more important significant risk factors are unsafe neighbourhoods, access to unhealthy food, limited access to recreational facilities or parks, low socioeconomic status, unhealthy social environment, unsafe water, sanitation and low hygiene, poor quality of air (WHO 2017b).

BOX 3.3 Risk factor

A risk factor is any attribute, characteristic or exposure of an individual that increases the likelihood of developing a disease or injury (WHO 2017b).

With the purpose of designing healthy built environments and taking into account previous definitions (WHO 2017b), the term "**health risk factor in built environments**" is defined:

BOX 3.4 Health risk factors in built environments

Health risk factors in built environments are all risk factors that are present in built environments, namely living and working environments, indoors or outdoors. A given exposure or series of exposures to them may have damaged or will damage the health of individuals. For example, increased noise levels and lack of daylight in a built environment are parameters in the group of physical risks factors; formaldehyde, phthalates in the air are parameters in the group of chemical health risk factors. Therefore, identification of health risks factors and their parameters in built environments is the key activity for effective control and prevention of health.

The standard CAN/CSA-Z1002-12 (2017)—Occupational health and safety—Hazard identification and elimination and risk assessment and control uses the following epidemiological terms: harm—"physical injury or damage to health" (CAN/CSA-Z1002-12 2017) and hazard: "a potential source of harm to a worker" (CAN/CSA-Z1002-12 2017).

Identification of health hazards and risk factors in built environments is a key activity for effective control and prevention against them and is the first step in a process called **health risk assessment (HRA)**. The Centers for Disease Control and Prevention (CDC 2009) define an HRA as: "a systematic approach to collecting information from individuals that identifies risk factors, provides individualized feedback, and links the person with at least one intervention to promote health, sustain function and/or prevent disease."

BOX 3.5 Health risk assessment

Health risk assessment is the process of estimating the nature and probability of adverse health effects in humans who may be exposed to chemicals in contaminated environmental media, now or in the future (EPA 2016).

The EPA uses health risk assessments to characterize the nature and magnitude of health risks to human beings (e.g., residents, workers, recreational visitors) and ecological receptors (e.g., birds, fish, wildlife) from chemical contaminants and other stressors that may be present in the environment.

The main steps of HRA (HSA 2017) for the prevention and control of health risk factors in built environments:

- **Identification of hazards and risk factors** that have the potential to cause harm (hazard identification) to humans and/or ecological systems regarding health.
- **Analysis and evaluation** of the risk in association with that hazard (risk analysis, and risk evaluation). Which includes:

- **Dose-Response Assessment**: relationship between exposure and effects
- **Exposure Assessment**: frequency, timing, and levels of contact with the potential hazard
- **Risk Characterization**: summary of an overall conclusion about risk, how well the data support conclusions about the nature and extent of the risk from exposure to potential hazard

- **Determining appropriate ways to eliminate** the hazard, or control the risk when the hazard cannot be eliminated (risk control).

Risk control includes actions that can be taken to reduce the exposure to the potential hazard. Alternatively, the control could be implemented to remove the hazard or to reduce the likelihood of the risk by reducing the exposure to that hazard (HSA 2017). Actions are listed hierarchically from the most preferred to least preferred (1–6):

1. **Elimination** of the hazards (e.g., removal of dangerous substance from construction materials),
2. **Substitution** of the hazards with those of lower risk (e.g., usage of less toxic substitutes),
3. **Isolation** of the hazard (e.g., noise-isolated room for noisy equipment),
4. **Engineering approaches** to the hazards (e.g., redesigning a process to place a barrier between the person and the hazard),
5. **Administrative approaches** to the hazards (e.g., adopting safe work practices, training to reduce the potential for harm and/or adverse health effects to people),
6. **Usage of personal protective equipment**.

In the framework of HRA, health risk factors and their main parameters in built environments are identified and classified in Sect. 3.2.

3.2 Identification and Classification of Health Risk Factors in Built Environments and Their Parameters

During the time spent indoors, people are exposed to numerous health risk factors, exposure to which can affect human health. The extent of the effects depends on their exposure dose, exposure time, type of pollutants, and people's individual characteristics (Yassi et al. 2001). Health risk factors in built environments can be classified in various ways, according to the purpose of classification. The most common classification of health risk factors was defined in the book on "Basic Environmental Health" by Yassi et al. (2001):

- **Biological risk factors**,
- **Chemical risk factors**,
- **Physical risk factors**, and
- **Psychosocial, personal and other risk factors**.

Table 3.2 Classified health risk factors in built environments with their main parameters (Kukec and Dovjak 2014; Dovjak and Kukec 2014)

Biological	Chemical	Physical	Psychosocial	Personal	Others
– Moulds – Bacteria – Microbes volatile organic compounds – House dust	– Construction and household products – Formaldehyde – Phthalates – Man-made mineral fibres – Volatile organic compounds – Odours – Environmental tobacco smoke – Other indoor air pollutants	– Environmental parameters of thermal comfort – Parameters related to building ventilation – Noise, vibrations – Daylight – Electromagnetic fields – Ions – Ergonomics – Universal design	– Occupational stress – Social status – Loneliness, helplessness – Work organization, communication, supervision	– Gender – Individual characteristics, health status	– Location, geo-pathogenic zones – Building characteristics – Ownership – Presence of insect, rodents, use of insecticide, disinfection, rat-killing products

On the basis of a comprehensive systematic literature review of 96 scientific articles published between 1974 and 2014 (Kukec and Dovjak 2014; Dovjak and Kukec 2014), key parameters within every group of health risk factors are identified and classified (Table 3.2).

In Sects. 3.3–3.7, detailed determinants of health risk factors and their main parameters are provided, followed by the results of epidemiological studies proving the association between potential health outcomes and health risk factors in built environments.

3.3   Association Between Potential Health Outcomes and Physical Health Risk Factors in Built Environments

The most researched parameters in the group of physical risk factors in built environments are those of thermal comfort, building ventilation, noise, vibration, daylight, electromagnetic fields, ions, as well as ergonomic issues and universal design. Deviations of one or several physical health risk factors from the optimal values may result in various health outcomes.

> **Environmental parameters of thermal comfort** and thermal stress are physical quantities connected with the environment: air temperature, mean radiant temperature, absolute air humidity, air velocity and surface temperature (ISO 7726: 1998). In addition to environmental parameters, metabolic rate and clothing also have a direct impact on a person's perception of thermal comfort.

Environmental parameters of thermal comfort that deviate from optimal values result in uncomfortable or even in unhealthy conditions (Prek and Butala 2012). Studies show that general dissatisfaction with the **indoor air temperature** and **indoor air humidity** may be related to the increase of SBS (Sick Building Syndrome) symptoms (Valbjorn and Kousgaard 1986; Valbjorn and Skov 1987). Jaakkola et al. (1989) carried out a study in a modern eight-floor office building in Finland (N = 2,150 workers) and found a linear correlation between the amount of SBS symptoms, sensation of dryness, and a rise in **air temperature** above 22 °C. SBS symptoms increased both when the indoor air temperature was considered to be too cold and too warm.

Nordström et al. (1994) performed a study in new and well-ventilated geriatric hospital units in southern Sweden (N = 104 employees). It was stated that in Scandinavia, the **indoor relative humidity** in well-ventilated buildings in winter was usually in the range between 10 and 35%, which resulted in increased numbers of dissatisfied persons. It was concluded that air **humidification** during the **heating**

season in colder climates can decrease the symptoms of SBS and the perception of dry air among employees. Lim et al. (2015) studied the association between SBS symptoms and some potential risk factors in an office environment (selected personal factors, office characteristics and indoor office exposures) among office workers (N = 695) from a Malaysian university. The weekly prevalence of dermal, mucosal and general symptoms of SBS was 11.9%, 16.0% and 23.0%, respectively. The SBS symptoms occurring among the workers in the offices were associated with low **relative air humidity** (p = 0.04; the association was statistically significant) and high **air temperature** in the office (p = 0.05; the association was statistically significant). Andersen et al. (1974) performed an experiment in a climate chamber, in which eight healthy young men were exposed to clean dry air with a temperature of 23 °C. The experiment showed that very low **indoor relative humidity** (less than 20%) can cause drying of the mucous membranes and of the skin in some individuals.

BOX 3.6 p-value (probability)

The probability that a test statistic would be as extreme as observed or more extreme if the null hypothesis were true. Letter p stands for this probability. Investigators may arbitrarily set their own significance levels, but in most biomedical and epidemiological works, a study result in which the p-value is less than 5% (p < 0.05) or 1% (p < 0.01) is considered sufficiently unlikely to have occurred by chance to justify the designation "statistically significant" (Porta 2008).

BOX 3.7 Relative risk (RR) and Odds ratio (OR)

RR is the ratio between the risk of an event among the exposed and the risk among the unexposed; this usage is synonymous with risk ratio. **OR** is a measure of association between an exposure and an outcome. The OR represents the odds that an outcome will occur given a particular exposure, compared to the odds of the outcome occurring in the absence of that exposure. OR/RR = 1 Exposure does not affect the odds of outcome; OR/RR > 1 Exposure associated with higher odds of outcome; OR/RR < 1 Exposure associated with lower odds of outcome (Porta 2008).

High **indoor air humidity** usually appears in buildings located in a hot-humid climate. However, higher indoor relative humidity (more than 80%) may also occur in other buildings, especially due to incorrectly designed building envelopes, systems and installations, processes of increased steam production, water damage, and flooding. These conditions may lead to dampness, stuffy odour, visible mould, and adverse health effects. Dampness may be a strong predictor of SBS symptoms. Li et al. (1997) evaluated the association between measures of **dampness** and symptoms of respiratory illness in 612 employees in 56 day-care centres in the Taipei, Taiwan area. Dampness was found in 75.3% of the centres, visible mould in 25.8%, stuffy odour in 50.0%, water damage in 49.3%, and flooding in 57.2%. Furthermore, the prevalence of SBS symptoms in the day-care workers was statistically significant among those who worked in centres that had mould or dampness.

Additionally, lower **surface temperatures** may result in local discomfort, radiative asymmetry, and water condensation. Studies made by Barna and Bánhidi (2012) showed that low **surface temperatures** often result in thermally uncomfortable conditions and the higher prevalence of SBS symptoms. Amin et al. (2015) investigated thermal conditions and SBS symptoms in three air-conditioned engineering education laboratories located at University Tun Hussein Onn Malaysia (N = 71 undergraduate and postgraduate students). The results show that the **mean radiant temperature** was not within the recommended range (minimum 17.8 °C, maximum 22.42 °C). A subjective measurement with questionnaire surveys was also performed. Among the symptoms present due to unacceptable thermal conditions in all laboratories, dry skin was the most common (40.85%), followed by runny nose (31%), dry eyes (29.58%), blocked/stuffy nose (28.17%), tiredness (26.76%) and flu-like symptoms (21.13%).

Inadequate ventilation is associated with the accumulation of a variety of pollutants from building materials and indoor activities, dampness, and with a higher risk of airborne infectious disease transmission among the occupants. Identifying and controlling common indoor air pollutants can protect human health.

The general purpose of **ventilation in buildings** is to provide healthy air for breathing by diluting the pollutants originating from the building itself and activities performed in the building and removing the pollutants from it (Awbi 2003).

Norhidayah et al. (2013) studied the association between **indoor air quality (IAQ) parameters** and symptoms of SBS in three selected buildings. The findings suggested that important predictors of sick building syndromes are **ventilation** and the accumulation of possible contaminants within the indoor environment. Other studies emphasized that the main causes for the SBS symptoms related to building ventilation are **inadequate functioning, obsolete** and **inadequately maintained HVAC systems, decreased number of air changes** and **decreased volume of clean air** (ECA 1989). A literature review of 41 studies (Seppänen et al. 1999) showed that **ventilation rates** below 10 L/s per person in office buildings were associated with statistically significant worsening in one or more health or perceived air quality outcomes. Some studies determined that increases in **ventilation rates** up to approximately 20 L/s per person were associated with significant decreases in the prevalence of the SBS symptoms or with significant improvements in perceived IAQ. The reviewed studies reported RR of 1.5–2.0 for respiratory illnesses and RR of 1.1–6.0 for the SBS symptoms for low compared to high ventilation rates.

A literature review by Carrer et al. (2015) estimated the minimum **ventilation rates** for which no effects on some health outcomes were observed. The lowest ventilation rates for which no adverse effects were seen for respiratory symptoms, asthma or allergy symptoms, airborne infectious diseases or acute health symptoms (SBS/BR symptoms) were about 6–7 L/s per person. In terms of effects on short-term absence rates and performance and learning, these minimum rates are much higher, ranging from 16–24 L/s per person. If the lowest ventilation rates for which no adverse effects were seen were selected based on building type, then the ventilation rates in homes and dormitories would be 6–7 L/s per person, in schools 12 L/s per person and in offices 25 L/s per person.

Numerous researchers have examined the prevalence of SBS symptoms in naturally ventilated and air-conditioned buildings. A literature review on the ventilation of office buildings (Seppänen and Fisk 2002) indicated that occupants of **naturally ventilated offices** had fewer SBS symptoms than occupants of **air-conditioned offices** did. A similar study was performed by Costa and Brickus (2000) in a central-air-conditioned shopping centre and in natural ventilated commercial shops in Rio de Janeiro, Brazil. Air-conditioned buildings were associated with increased SBS symptoms.

Noise is unwanted sound judged to be unpleasant, loud or disruptive to hearing (WHO 2013). Exposure to noise in built environments has several harmful impacts on health: disturbed sleep, cardiovascular and psychophysiological effects, and reduced performance, as well as provoking annoyance responses and changes in social behaviour.

Excessive noise seriously harms human health and interferes with people's daily activities (WHO 2013). Wonga (2009) studied the prevalence of SBS among apartment residents of 748 households in Hong Kong. The major indoor environmental quality problem perceived by the residents was **noise**. In addition to **excessive noise, low-frequency noise** (20–100 Hz) may also cause health problems. Low-frequency noise is found in buildings with industrial machines or ventilation machinery. Certain body organs, specifically the eyes, have characteristic resonance frequencies in the range of 1–20 Hz (ECA 1989). Hodgson et al. (1987) observed that irritability and dizziness experienced by a group of secretaries working in new offices correlated significantly with the **vibrations** measured on their desks. The vibrations were caused by an adjacent pump room.

Lighting in buildings, especially **daylight**, should be designed for the visual needs of the users and their expected tasks within a given active space as well as non-visual effects (Webb 2006).

Many studies have found some potential health consequences due to a **lack of daylight** in built environments. Nicklas and Bailey (1997) performed some analyses of the performance of students in daylit schools. They compared two groups of students from elementary schools in Alberta, Canada: the first group attending a school with **full-spectrum light**, the second group attending a similar school with **normal lighting conditions**. The results showed that the first group of students were healthier and attended school 3.2–3.8 days more per year; full-spectrum light induced more positive moods in students. Because of the additional vitamin D received by the students in the first group, they had 9 times less dental decay, and they were 2.1 cm higher compared to students in the second group.

The health benefits of **daylight** have also been demonstrated in healthcare facilities. Benedetti et al. (2001) investigated the effect of **direct sunlight** in the morning on the length of hospitalization of depressed bipolar patients. The length of hospitalization was recorded for a sample of 415 unipolar and 187 depressed bipolar patients, assigned to rooms with eastern or western windows. Bipolar patients exposed to direct sunlight in the morning had on average 3.67-day shorter hospital stays than patients in western rooms. No effect was found in unipolar patients. A similar study was performed by Beauchemin and Hays (1996). Patients in **sunny rooms** had on average 2.6-day (15%) shorter stays compared to those in dull rooms. Heerwagen (1986) found that patients with a **view of trees** had better post-surgical recovery, while patients in the same hospital with **a view of a brick wall** stayed longer, took more narcotic analgesics, and had more post-surgical complications. Choi et al. (2012) studied the effect of daylight on patients' average length of hospital stay. They compared different **orientations of patient rooms** in each ward of the general hospital in Incheon, Korea. The results showed 16–41% shorter hospital stay in wards with optimal daylight conditions. Daylight also has an important role in curative and preventive medicine. Terman et al. (1986) claimed that improved **interior lighting** could reduce the common subclinical problems, such as oversleeping, overeating, energy loss, and work disturbance. Light can help cure rickets, osteomalacia, and Seasonal Affective Disorder (SAD).

Lack of daylight in built environments has adverse health effects on human health and their determinants. Daylight has been associated with improved mood and enhanced morale (Robbins 1986). Clark and Watson (1988) found that negative moods are associated with discomfort and distraction, whereas positive moods are associated with the physical setting at work and daily activities, such as social interactions among employees, which often results in lower absenteeism rates. Markussen and Røed (2014) examined the impact of hours of daylight on sick-leave absences among workers in Norway. They found that each additional hour of daylight increases the daily entry rate to absenteeism by 0.5% and the corresponding recovery rate by 0.8%. The overall relationship between absenteeism and **daylight hours** was negative.

Nicklas and Bailey (1997) investigated the relationships between elementary and middle school student performance in North Carolina and natural daylighting. The results showed that the students who attended daylit schools outperformed those attending non-daylit schools by 5–14%. Moreover, children under **electric lights** throughout the day showed decreased mental capabilities, agitated physical behaviour, and fatigue (Hathaway et al. 1992). Abdel-Hamid et al. (2013) carried out a cross-sectional study at the Faculty of Medicine, Ain Shams University, Cairo, Egypt. The results of the self-administered questionnaire with 826 workers showed that fatigue and headache were the most prevalent symptoms related to SBS (76.9 and 74.7%). **Poor lighting, lack of sunlight** and **absence of air currents** were associated statistically with SBS symptoms and were affected also by other parameters: **poor ventilation, high noise, temperature, humidity, environmental tobacco smoke, use of photocopiers, and inadequate office cleaning**.

In the framework of a WHO workshop on Electromagnetic Hypersensitivity it was described as: "sensitivity to **electromagnetic field** (EMF) that comprises nervous system symptoms like headache, fatigue, stress, sleep disturbances, skin symptoms like prickling, burning sensations and rashes, pain and ache in muscles and many other health problems" (WHO 2004, p. V).

Related to adverse health effects due to exposure to **electromagnetic** fields (EMF), many articles have been published over the years. A recent in-depth review of the scientific literature, WHO (2014), concluded that current evidence did not confirm the existence of any health consequences from exposure to low-level EMF. Exposures to higher levels that might be harmful are restricted by national and international guidelines. However, a number of epidemiological studies (WHO 2014) suggest small increases in risk of childhood leukaemia with exposure to **low-frequency magnetic fields** at home. Some individuals reported "hypersensitivity" to **electric or magnetic fields**. Eriksson and Stenberg (2006) investigated the prevalence of general, mucosal, and skin symptoms in the Swedish population (N = 3,000, age 18–64). The survey addressed 25 symptoms, principally general, mucosal, and skin symptoms. The SBS symptoms, skin symptoms and symptoms similar to those reported by individuals with "electric hypersensitivity" were significantly more prevalent among employees who used display screen equipment extensively.

Small **air ions** are electrically charged clusters consisting of atmospheric molecules or atoms that have lost or gained electrons to impart a net **positive or negative charge**. Atmospheric space charge in the form of small **air ions** may be generated from natural sources, such as changes in atmospheric and weather conditions, including rain, wind, and snow, as well as natural radioactivity in geological formations, cosmic radiation, waterfalls, and combustion processes (Alexander et al. 2013).

Researchers (ILO 2011; Reilly and Stevenson 1993) support the view that **negative ions** have a positive effect on health, including improved mood, stabilized catecholamine regulation and circadian rhythm, enhanced recovery from physical exertion and protection from positive ion-related stress and exhaustion disorders. The minimum acceptable concentration of negative ions for indoor air is 200–300 ions per cm^3. The optimal level is 1000–1500 negative ions per cm^3 (Jokl 1989). The lack of negative ions in the air may be responsible for SBS (ECA 1989). Bowers et al. (2018) evaluated the effectiveness of 30- and 60-minute daily exposure to high-density compared to zero-density (placebo condition) negative air ions over 18 days on the symptoms of seasonal affective disorder (SAD) in 40 participants under controlled laboratory conditions. The results showed that exposure to negative air ions significantly improved winter depression symptoms. All sources of fire (Sulman 1980a, b), and especially cigarette smoking (Jokl 1989), electrical radiators, and air-conditioners increase the concentration of **positive ions**, which may be related to SBS. According to Sulman (1980a, b), the reported physiological effects of positive ions include inhibited cell tissue culture growth, increased respiratory rate, increased basal metabolism, increased blood pressure, headache, fatigue, nausea, nasal obstructions, sore throat, dizziness and increased skin temperatures. The researchers found that the electrical charges (positive ionization) engendered by approaching weather fronts produce the release of serotonin and weather sensitivity reactions (irritation syndrome, exhaustion syndrome, hyperthyroidism) (Sulman 1980a, b). One way to increase the level of negative ions in indoor environments is a water fountain or live plants (which must be non-toxic). Plants can also be used for phytoremediation, the removal of toxins from the air to ameliorate indoor air quality. The ability of species to remove benzene, formaldehyde, and other indoor air pollutants has been proven by studies (Liu et al. 2007; Aydogan and Montoya 2011).

Ergonomics is the science of matching the job to the worker and the product to the user (Pheasant 1991, p. 3). The main approach of ergonomics is in user-centred design: "If a product (environment or system) is intended for human use, then its design should be based on the characteristics of its human users" (Pheasant 1986, 1987).

Principles of user-centred design are combined in universal design.

Universal Design is a design and composition of an environment, which can be accessed, understood and used to the greatest extent possible by all people regardless of their age, size, ability or disability. An environment (or any building, product or service in that environment) should be designed to meet the needs of all people who use it. This is not a special requirement from which only a minority of the population benefits, but a fundamental condition of good design (NDA 2014).

Hedge and Erickson (1998) define that worker ergonomics (designing the work/environment/process/equipment to fit the worker, instead of forcing the worker to fit the work/environment/process/equipment) and issues of universal design (barrier-free environment for all groups of functional disabilities) (Dovjak and Kristl 2009) also involves significant physical risk factors that have to be considered for the prevention of SBS.

3.4 Association Between Potential Health Outcomes and Chemical Health Risk Factors in Built Environments

The most important chemical risk factors affecting health are construction and household products and emitted pollutants from furniture and equipment, especially formaldehyde, phthalates, volatile organic compounds, odours, environmental tobacco smoke, biocides, and others. According Simmons and Richard (1997), many **construction products** used for waterproofing, insulating, fireproofing, roofing, painting, plastering, building and treating floors, as well as surface coatings, contain toxic chemicals.

The first epidemiological studies of cancer risk in relation to exposure to **asbestos** were reported in the 1950s (Marsili et al. 2016). Until the late 1970s, **asbestos** was used in construction products such as asbestos insulation, roofing, flooring, adhesives, duct connectors as well as protective clothing, household items, and others. All types of asbestos cause lung cancer, mesothelioma, cancer of the larynx and ovary, and asbestosis (fibrosis of the lungs) (WHO 2017c). According to Commission Directive (1999), all EU Member States banned asbestos in 2005. Consequently, for countries that have stopped using asbestos, their asbestos-related disease burden will most likely decrease (Kameda et al. 2014). Nevertheless, the EU currently carries the largest share of the global asbestos-related disease burden as a consequence of heavy asbestos use in previous decades.

European countries that adopt the EU REACH regulation restrict the use and sale of certain **specific lead compounds for use in paints** (UNEP 2016). Nevertheless, in many countries, architectural/decorative paints still contain significant concentrations of lead (Gottesfeld 2015). Childhood lead poisoning has been a recognized clinical entity since the first decade of the 20th century, when leaded petrol and lead-based paints were common (WHO 2010).

Many new chemicals have not yet been tested for their impact on human health, which presents a problem (Petrović 2017). The problem of exponential increase in the development of synthetic and petroleum-based chemicals since World War II was highlighted by Petrović (2017). The problem is even more serious in case of numerous emission sources, such as **radon emission from constructional complexes** (i.e., fly ash bricks) and **from soils and rock** (Chauhan et al. 2003). The exposure of people to high concentrations of radon and its isotopes for an extended period leads to pathological effects, such as functional respiratory changes and the occurrence of lung cancer (EPA 2017a).

Throughout their life cycle construction products may emit harmful substances in the surrounding environment (Šestan et al. 2013; Dovjak and Kristl 2011). To provide good indoor air quality (IAQ), holistic measures with step-by-step activities have to be performed (i.e., including actions on location-building/constructional complexes-system). At the first stage of design, it is important to perform source control measures with the selection of non-toxic construction products. Moreover, some researchers have also studied so-called sorptive building material as an effective method for improving IAQ. Park et al. (2015) proved the effect of concentration reduction through the use of sorptive building materials in office areas.

In addition to construction products, **household products** also have to be considered from the aspects of IAQ. For example, the use of air-fresheners may be related to poor indoor air quality and may lead to SBS symptoms and other adverse health effects (NIPH 2009; Zock et al. 2007; Cohen et al. 2007). Within the follow-up of the European Community Respiratory Health Survey in 10 countries, Zock et al. (2007) identified 3,503 persons without asthma, who were regularly cleaning their homes. The results showed that the use of **cleaning sprays** at least once a week (42% of participants) was associated with the incidence of asthma symptoms or medication and wheeze. The incidence of physician-diagnosed asthma was higher among those who used sprays at least 4 days per week. Dose-response relationships were apparent for the frequency of use and the number of different sprays.

Moreover, due to low air humidity in buildings, humidifiers are often used. **Humidifiers** in the ventilation circuit provide a source of microbes to flourish, and also provide a reason for adding biocides to humidified water. Many of these **biocides** are irritants or allergens (Burge 2004). These products are highly irritant in concentrated form; when dispersed in the indoor atmosphere, at low concentrations, they may cause mucous membrane irritation in susceptible individuals (Burge 2004).

Construction products and wooden furniture (e.g., plywood, particleboard, fibreboard, OSB, panel boards, urea-formaldehyde foam), paints, adhesives, varnishes, floor finishes, disinfectants, cleaning agents and other household products emit **formaldehyde (HCHO)** (Šestan et al. 2013).

The results of several studies of indoor/outdoor ratios of **formaldehyde** in buildings range approximately from 3 to 18 (ARB 2012; Blondel and Plaisance

2011; Sakai et al. 2004). Formaldehyde may be the cause of SBS, because it irritates both the eyes, as well as the upper and lower respiratory tract. It may also be responsible for allergic disorders, including asthma (Hendrick and Lane 1977). In a study among students in schools in Malaysia (N = 462 pupils), formaldehyde and other selected indoor air pollutants were associated with rhinitis, ocular, nasal and dermal symptoms, headache, and fatigue. Norbäck et al. (2017) arrived at similar findings. Formaldehyde was associated with ocular (p = 0.004), throat symptoms (p = 0.006) and fatigue (p = 0.001).

Šestan et al. (2013) reviewed 11 epidemiological studies that monitored the concentrations of **formaldehyde** in buildings (nine studies on residential buildings and two studies on public buildings). They found that the measured concentrations of formaldehyde ranged from 0.0016 ppm (2 $\mu g/m^3$) to 0.109 ppm (134 $\mu g/m^3$). The measured concentrations from the reviewed studies may cause irritation of the upper respiratory tract in the exposed individuals. An examination of studies (2005 and more recent studies) (Salthammer et al. 2010) indicated that under normal living conditions the average exposure to formaldehyde seems to lie between 0.0163 ppm (20 $\mu g/m^3$) and 0.0326 ppm (40 $\mu g/m^3$). Salthammer et al. (2010) also emphasized that new buildings with changed microclimate conditions may exhibit higher average and maximum concentrations, which may lead to the increased exposures and health risks, particularly in the group of sensitive individuals.

> **Polyvinyl chloride (PVC)** construction products usually contain plasticisers, **phthalate esters** that may be emitted from PVC during the whole life cycle of the product. PVC materials are problematic during normal use of the building or during emergency situations (i.e., fire).

A comprehensive literature review by Dovjak and Kristl (2011) indicated that the use of PVC construction products in indoor environments may have adverse health effects. **Phthalates** are thought to be responsible for low testosterone levels, declining sperm counts and quality, genital malformations, retarded sexual development or even reproductive abnormalities and increased incidences of certain types of cancer (Heudorf et al. 2007). Epidemiological studies (Jaakkola et al. 1999; Bornehag et al. 2004) state that the presence of PVC flooring and walls is related to asthma, rhinitis, wheeze, cough, phlegm, nasal congestion, nasal excretion and eczema in children. These findings underscore the need to consider the health aspects of materials used in indoor environments.

A systematic review and meta-analysis of 14 laboratory toxicology studies in adults (1950–2007) assessed the relationship between PVC-related occupational exposure (meat wrappers, hospital and office workers, firefighters, PVC processors) and the risk of asthma, allergies, or related respiratory effects (Jaakkola and Knight 2008).

In the study by Subedi et al. (2017), the concentrations of potentially toxic **plasticizers** (phthalates and non-phthalates) were investigated in 28 dust samples collected from three different indoor environments (e.g., homes, salons, and day-care centres) across the USA. The estimated daily intakes of **total phthalates** (n = 7) for children and toddlers through indoor dust in childcare facilities were 1.6 times higher than the non-phthalate plasticizers (n = 3), whereas the estimated daily intake of total non-phthalates for all age groups in the domestic environment was 1.9 times higher than the phthalate plasticizers. This study reveals a more elevated (∼3 fold) occupational intake of phthalate and non-phthalate plasticizers through the indoor dust at hair salons compared to domestic environments in the USA.

During emergency situations (e.g., in case of fire), hazardous products such as **carbon monoxide, carbon dioxide, hydrogen chloride, hydrochloric acid, dioxins, smoke/soot,** etc. may form (Dovjak and Kristl 2011).

Phthalates can be adsorbed onto indoor surfaces (carpet, wood, and skin) and re-emitted in the indoor air (Xu et al. 2009).

Man-made mineral fibre (MMMF) is a generic name used to describe an inorganic fibrous material manufactured primarily from glass, rock, minerals, slag and processed inorganic oxides. According to the International Agency for Research on Cancer (IARC 2002), MMMF is classified into five categories: continuous glass filament, glass wool (insulation wool and special purpose wool), rock wool, slag wool, refractory ceramic and other.

According to the results of epidemiological studies, **MMMFs** have adverse health effects (EC 2012). Acoustic ceilings may contain MMMF that may be transferred from such surfaces to skin and eyes, normally by direct hand contact. However, MMMF may also be transferred via air transmission modes. Nielsen (1987) proved that especially high concentrations may be found in rooms with uncovered ceilings, but also in rooms where the fibres are bound by a water-soluble glue and exposed to water damage. **Unsealed fibreglass** and **other insulation** material lining the ventilation ducts can release particulate material into the air. Such material can also become wet, creating an ideal and often concealed growth medium for microorganisms (Redlich et al. 1997).

Volatile organic compounds (VOCs) are emitted as gases from certain solids or liquids. VOCs include a variety of chemicals, some of which may have short and long-term adverse health effects. Sources of VOCs are household products (e.g., wood preservatives, aerosol sprays, cleansers and disinfectants, moth repellents and air fresheners, stored fuels and automotive products, hobby supplies, dry-cleaned clothing, pesticide) and other products (building materials and furnishings, office equipment) (EPA 2017b).

Volatile organic compounds (VOCs) are suspected to be one of the major causes of SBS (Nakaoka et al. 2014; Yu and Kim 2012; Logue et al. 2011; Takigawa et al. 2009; Wang et al. 2007; Mølhave 2003; Schneider et al. 2003; Hodgson 2002; Wolkoff 1987). Construction products, furniture, household products (waxes, detergent, insecticides), products of personal hygiene (cosmetics), do-it-yourself goods (resins), office materials (photocopier ink) or environmental tobacco smoke (ETS) are all sources of VOCs in indoor environments. Wolkoff (1987) found that concentrations of VOCs depend on the type of the room, activity and time. **VOCs** may affect human health and can sometimes also be the source of **odours** (ECA 1989). Takigawa et al. (2009) conducted a study in residential buildings in Okayama, Japan (N = 86 men, 84 women). The results showed that **aldehyde** levels in indoor air increased frequently and markedly in the newly diseased and ongoing SBS groups. About 10% of subjects suffered from SBS in 2004 and 2005. Similar findings were made by Takigawa et al. (2012). They studied 871 people living in 260 single-family houses in 2004 and 2005. Approximately 14 and 12% of subjects were identified as having SBS in the first and second years, respectively. Elevated levels of indoor **aldehydes** and **aliphatic hydrocarbons** in indoor air increased the possible risk of SBS to occur in residents living in new houses. Goodman et al. (2017) systematically evaluated 25 years (1991–2016) of investigations of VOC presence in Australian indoor environments. New homes had the highest VOC levels among all studies of domestic housing. Concentrations of nearly all pollutants were several times higher indoor compared to outdoor. **Terpenes (d-limonene** and **α-pinene)** were among the most indoor prevalent compounds.

> **Odours** are organic or inorganic compounds that originate from within a building, or they can be drawn into a building from the outdoors. Indoor odour sources are usually associated with construction products, household products, furnishings, office equipment, insufficient ventilation, problems with mould, bio-effluents, etc. Odours are a significant source of indoor environmental quality problems in buildings (CDC 2013).

According to the Report of the European Commission on SBS ECA (1989), the **hidden olfs** (a unit used to measure the strength of a pollution source) from materials and systems are claimed to be one of the major reasons for SBS. Nakaoka et al. (2014) examined the correlation between the sum of VOCs, total odour threshold ratio, and SBS symptoms. The findings indicated that the **total odour threshold ratio** and the concentration of VOCs were correlated with SBS symptoms among sensitive people. Wang et al. (2013) studied the prevalence of **perceptions of odours** and sensations of air humidity and SBS symptoms in domestic environments. Parents (N = 4,530) of 1-to-8-year-old children from randomly selected kindergartens in Chongqing, China participated. Stuffy odours, unpleasant odour, pungent odour, mould odour, tobacco smoke odour, humid air and dry air in the preceding three months (weekly or sometimes) was reported by 31.4%, 26.5%, 16.1%, 10.6%, 33.0%, 32.1% and 37.2% of the parents, respectively. The prevalence of parents regarding SBS symptoms was: 78.7% for general symptoms, 74.3% for mucosal symptoms, and 47.5% for skin symptoms. Multi-nominal regression analyses for associations between odours/sensations of air humidity and SBS symptoms showed that the odds ratio for "weekly" SBS symptoms was consistently higher than for "sometimes" SBS symptoms.

Environmental tobacco smoke (ETS) is composed of both mainstream and side-stream smoke. ETS usually contains more than 4,000 different chemicals. Undiluted side-stream smoke contains higher concentrations of several chemicals than the mainstream smoke inhaled by the smoker. These chemicals include 2-naphthylamine, N-nitrosodimethylamine, 4-aminobiphenyl, and carbon monoxide (CCOHS 2011). The side-stream smoke may even be more of an irritant than the mainstream smoke (ECA 1989).

ETS is one of the main causes of SBS symptoms (CCOHS 2011). Studies on the correlations between **ETS exposure** and SBS showed that SBS was statistically more pronounced in smokers than in non-smokers (Valbjorn and Skov 1987) and there was an increase of symptoms in non-smokers and ex-smokers exposed to ETS in comparison to the same non-exposed categories (Robertson et al. 1988). Mizoue et al. (2001) analysed the data from a 1998 cross-sectional survey of 1,281 municipal employees who worked in a variety of buildings in a Japanese city. Among non-smokers, the odds ratio for the association between SBS and 4 h of **ETS exposure** per day was 2.7, and for most symptom categories, the odds ratios increased with increasing hours of ETS exposure. Working overtime (for 30 or more hours per month) was also associated with SBS symptoms, but the crude odds ratio of 3.0 for SBS was reduced by 21% after adjustment of variables associated with overtime work and by 49% after further adjustment of perceived work overload.

CO_2 is one of the most important indicators for indoor air quality and adequacy of building ventilation. The main indoor source of CO_2 in most buildings is human metabolic activity.

In terms of worker safety, Occupational Safety and Health Administration (OSHA) set a permissible exposure limit (PEL) for CO_2 of 5,000 parts per million (ppm) over an eight-hour workday. Similarly, the American Conference of Governmental Industrial Hygienists (ACGIH) defined the TLV (threshold limit value) as 5,000 ppm for an eight-hour workday, with a ceiling exposure limit of 30,000 ppm for a 10-minute period based on acute inhalation data (NIOSH 1976).

For the design and assessment of energy performance in buildings, recommended CO_2 concentrations above outdoor concentration are defined by EN 1525 (2007). For example, for a Category I environment, the recommended CO_2 concentration for energy calculations and required control is 350 ppm above outdoors. ANSI/ASHRAE Standard 62.1 (2004) defines that CO_2 concentration should not exceed 2500 ppm, while 1000 ppm is the recommended value.

According to national Rules on the ventilation and air-conditioning of buildings (OJ RS No. 42/2002, 105/2002), the permissible value of CO_2 in indoor air is 3000 mg/m^3 (1667 ppm). However, studies report that even lower levels of CO_2 concentrations, compared to these recommended or regulated concentrations, may lead to occupant dissatisfaction and decreased productivity (Bakó-Biró et al. 2007). For example, concentrations higher than 1000 ppm were associated with an increased percentage of dissatisfied occupants (ECA 1989). Especially high concentrations were detected in 24 school buildings in Slovenia (Butala and Novak 1999), where the maximal concentration of CO_2 was above 7198 mg/m^3 (4000 ppm).

Seppänen et al. (1999) reviewed 41 studies with over 60,000 subjects on the associations between ventilation rates and **CO_2 concentrations** in non-residential and non-industrial buildings (primarily offices) with health outcomes. The risk of the SBS symptoms continued to decrease significantly with decreasing CO_2 concentrations below 800 ppm. A similar conclusion was presented in the study by Erdmann et al. (2002), Apte et al. (2000) and Tsai et al. (2012). Erdmann et al. (2002) found that higher concentrations of CO_2 (workday time-averaged indoor minus outdoor CO_2 concentrations) were associated with an increased prevalence of certain mucous membrane and lower respiratory SBS symptoms. Even the highest CO_2 concentrations did not exceed 1000 ppm. Apte et al. (2000) evaluated the relationship between indoor CO_2 concentrations and the SBS symptoms in occupants from 41 U.S. office buildings. Results showed that dose-response relationship with odds ratios per 100 ppm CO_2 ranged from 1.2 to 1.5 for sore throat, nose/sinus, tight chest, and wheezing. Tsai et al. (2012) evaluated the SBS symptoms among 111 office workers in August and November 2003. The most common symptoms of the five SBS groups were eye irritation, nonspecific and upper respiratory symptoms. They also proved that workers exposed to indoor CO_2 levels greater than 800 ppm were likely to report eye irritation or upper respiratory symptoms more frequently.

From the public health perspective, an important association was found between different sources of exposure to indoor air and health effects. The systematic review included eight studies that found associations between asthma and high levels of PM, VOC and endotoxins (Erklavec et al. 2017). Norbäck et al. (2017) studied associations between **VOC, formaldehyde, nitrogen dioxide (NO_2)** and **CO_2** in schools in Malaysia (N = 462 pupils) and rhinitis, ocular, nasal and dermal symptoms, headache and fatigue among students. The prevalences of weekly rhinitis, ocular, throat and dermal symptoms were 18.8%, 11.6%, 15.6%, and 11.1%, respectively. In total, 20.6% of students had weekly headaches and 22.1% fatigue. NO_2 was associated with ocular symptoms ($p < 0.001$) and fatigue (p = 0.01). Formaldehyde was associated with ocular (p = 0.004), throat symptoms (p = 0.006) and fatigue (p = 0.001). Xylene was associated with fatigue (p < 0.001), and benzaldehyde was associated with headache (p = 0.03). In conclusion, xylene, benzaldehyde, formaldehyde and NO_2 in schools can be risk factors for fatigue, ocular, and throat symptoms among students in Malaysia.

3.5   Association Between Potential Health Outcomes and Biological Health Risk Factors in Built Environments

Microorganisms are always present in our living space, but higher concentrations are a risk factor for the onset of various diseases, as they can affect people's well-being, work performance, and productivity, and trigger a number of negative effects on health. Microorganisms can have direct or indirect effects on the quality of our living space, health, and well-being. Building operation, ventilation, and occupancy drive the building microbiology. Buildings represent a good media for the growth of microorganisms (Adams et al. 2016).

Biological contaminants present in indoor air include bacteria, moulds, mildew, viruses, animal dander and cat saliva, house dust, mites, cockroaches, and pollen (EPA 2012). There are many indoor or outdoor sources of these pollutants (e.g., people, animals, soil, plant debris). Microbial pollution involves hundreds of species of bacteria and fungi that grow indoors when sufficient moisture is available. Exposure to microbial contaminants is associated with respiratory symptoms, allergies, asthma, and immunological reactions (WHO 2009c).

> **Mould** is all species of microscopic fungi that grow in the form of multicellular filaments, called hyphae. In contrast, microscopic fungi that grow as single cells are called yeasts. A connected network of tubular branching hyphae has multiple, genetically identical nuclei and is considered a single organism, referred to as a colony (Madigan and Martinko 2005).

The study by Straus (2009) emphasized the importance of **moulds** and their **mycotoxins** in the phenomenon of SBS. Zhang et al. (2012) studied the associations between dampness and indoor moulds in workplace buildings and selected biomarkers as well as incidence and remission of SBS. The study was based on a ten-year prospective study (1992–2002) in a random sample of adults (N = 429) from the Uppsala part of the European Community Respiratory Health Survey. Dampness was associated with increased incidence and decreased remission of SBS. **Dampness** and **moulds** increased bronchial responsiveness and eosinophilic inflammation. A similar study was performed by Sahlberg et al. (2013) in 159 homes of inhabitants in three EU cities (Reykjavik, Uppsala, Tartu). The associations between SBS, **microbial volatile organic compounds** (MVOC), and reports on dampness and mould were examined. The results showed that the indoor levels of some MVOCs were positively associated with SBS. Levels of **airborne moulds** and **bacteria** and some MVOCs were higher in dwellings with a history of dampness and moulds. Problems with dampness also exist in other environments, such as dorm rooms and schools. Sun et al. (2013) carried out a study in 1,569 dorm rooms in Tianjin, China (2006–2007; N = 3,712 students). A "mouldy odour" or "dry air" were perceived by occupants in 31% of dorm rooms. The adjusted odds ratio (AOR) of perceived mouldy odour for general SBS symptoms was 2.4, for mucosal symptoms 2.2, and for skin symptoms 2.0. Local mouldy odour around room corners or under radiators was reported by inspectors in 26% of dorm rooms. The study concluded that local mouldy odour perceived by inspectors was a significant risk factor for nose irritation (AOR 2.8).

BOX 3.8 Adjusted odds ratio (AOR)
Adjusted odds ratios (AOR) are most commonly used when the analysis includes several variables and takes into account the effect of all variables. Stratification and multiple regression techniques are two methods used to address confounding and produce "adjusted" ORs (Szumilas 2010).

Zhang et al. (2011) analysed the relationship between the concentration of **allergens** and **microbial compounds** and new onsets of SBS. The study was based on a two-year prospective analysis of pupils (N = 1,143) in a random sample of schools in China. The prevalence of mucosal and general symptoms was 33% and 28%, respectively, at baseline, and it increased during follow-up. At baseline, 27% reported at least one symptom that improved when pupils were away from school (school-related symptoms). The authors concluded that exposure to mould could increase the incidence of school-related symptoms.

Moulds as a consequent phenomenon of flooding were considered by a few studies. The review by Crook and Burton (2010) describes the role of moulds in SBS and BRI as a clinical condition with defined symptoms and signs in which the cause (aetiology) is building related and identifiable. In their study, they use as examples the after-effects of flooding in the UK in 2007, and Hurricane Katrina in the USA in 2005. These studies reported the health effects of exposure to moulds. Respiratory symptoms were positively correlated with exposure to water-damaged homes. Studies also concluded that respirators reduced symptoms when worn while in the water-damaged homes. The most commonly reported symptoms were nasal symptoms and cough.

Bacteria are defined as microscopic, single-celled organisms belonging to the Kingdom Monera that possess a prokaryotic type of cell structure, which means their cells are non-compartmentalized, and their DNA (usually circular) can be found throughout the cytoplasm rather than within a membrane-bound nucleus. Bacteria reproduce by fission or by forming spores. They can practically live everywhere. They can inhabit all kinds of environment, such as in soil, acidic hot springs, radioactive waste, seawater, deep in the Earth's crust, in the stratosphere, and even in the bodies of other organisms (Biology online 2017).

Teeuw et al. (1994) carried out a survey of SBS among 1,355 employees working in 19 governmental office buildings in the Netherlands. Physical, chemical, and microbiological characteristics between mechanically ventilated and naturally ventilated buildings were examined. Mechanically ventilated buildings were grouped as "healthy" or "sick" based on symptom prevalence (mean symptom prevalence <15% or >15 or = 15%). The authors found no differences in physical characteristics. However, the concentration of **airborne endotoxin** and **Gram-negative rods** were found in higher numbers in the "sick" mechanically ventilated buildings than in the "healthy" mechanically ventilated buildings and naturally ventilated buildings. The study concluded that airborne microbial contamination, in particular with Gram-negative rods and perhaps with **endotoxin**, may have a role in the causation of SBS.

Al-Hunaiti et al. (2017) analysed the **floor dust bacteria** and **fungi** and their coexistence with PAHs in Jordanian indoor environments (eight dwellings and an educational building) in Amman. The results showed that bacterial and fungal concentrations varied significantly among and within the tested indoor environments. Educational buildings have higher **Gram-negative bacteria** concentration than dwellings. **Gram −/+ bacteria** and **total fungal concentrations** were positively correlated.

Microbes volatile organic compounds (MVOCs) are a variety of volatile organic compounds formed in the primary and secondary metabolism of microorganisms (Korpi et al. 2009; Fu 2016). They are associated with mould and bacterial growth and responsible for the odorous smells (Ammann 1988). In total, around 1,200 MVOC have been identified, and around 250 MVOC from mould have been measured in indoor environmental studies (Fu 2016). The most obvious health effect of MVOC exposure is eye and upper-airway irritation (Korpi et al. 2009).

Araki et al. (2010) measured indoor **MVOC levels** in single-family homes and evaluated the relationship between exposure to them and SBS. The most frequently detected MVOC was 1-pentanol. Among 620 participants, 19.4% reported one or more mucous symptoms; irritation of the eyes, nose, airway, or coughing every week (weekly symptoms), and 4.8% reported that the symptoms were home-related. Weekly symptoms were not associated with any MVOC, whereas significant associations between home-related mucous symptoms and 1-octen-3-ol and 2-pentanol were obtained. Additionally, Sahlberg et al. (2013) examined whether MVOCs and airborne levels of bacteria, moulds, formaldehyde, and two plasticizers in dwellings were associated with the prevalence of SBS and studied associations between MVOCs and reports on dampness and mould. A total of 159 adults (57% females) participated (19% from Reykjavik, 40% from Uppsala, and 41% from Tartu). The results showed that MVOCs, such as 1-octen-3-ol, formaldehyde and the plasticizer Texanol, may be a risk factor for sick building syndrome. Moreover, concentrations of airborne moulds, bacteria and some other MVOCs were slightly higher in homes with reported dampness and mould. Some MVOCs may have adverse effects on respiratory, nervous, and circulatory systems and may have carcinogenic effects (Yu et al. 2009).

A case-control investigation by Choi et al. (2017) studies the association between MVOC and its risks on childhood asthma and allergies within damp homes (198 cases, 202 controls). Results showed that among the children who lived in high absolute humidity homes, a natural log (ln)-unit of total sum of 28 MVOCs was associated with 2.5-times greater odds of the case status (95% CI, 1.0–6.2; $p = 0.046$), compared to 0.7-times the odds (95% CI, 0.4–1.0; $p = 0.074$) of the same outcome among low absolute humidity homes. Specifically, joint exposure to high MVOCs and high absolute humidity was associated with 2.6-times greater odds of the doctor-diagnosed asthma status (95% CI, 0.7–8.91; $p = 0.137$).

BOX 3.9 Confidence interval (CI)

Confidence interval (CI) is a type of interval estimate (of a population parameter) that is computed from the observed data. It gives an estimated range of values which is likely to include an unknown population parameter, the estimated range being calculated from a given set of sample data (Easton and McColl 1997).

Pantoja et al. (2016) analysed the air quality of a public referral hospital in Fortaleza, Ceará, Brazil in terms of fungal volatile organic compounds (FVOCs), to establish ways to improve monitoring methods and control of specific sectors in the hospital. The results showed that 2-heptanone and 2-methyl-1-propanol were the most frequent FVOCs. Moreover, the climatic data showed the incidence of FVOCs regardless of the climatic season.

Dust in homes, offices, and other built environments contains various organic and inorganic matter (Hess-Kosa 2002). The quantity and composition of house dust vary greatly with seasonal and environmental factors and also depends upon the HVAC system, cleaning habits, occupant activities, etc.

Poor building service maintenance, poor cleaning or poor cleanability increases the prevalence of SBS (Burge et al. 1990). Nexo et al. (1983) demonstrated a correlation between the **organic dust content of carpets** (predominantly skin scales, bacteria, and moulds) and the symptoms of SBS. Among 12 employees, five had symptoms related to the workplace.

Dust often contains substances emitted from construction products (e.g., phthalate esters and other plasticisers emitted from PVC construction products). Many emitted substances may have significant health concerns. Kishi et al. (2012) performed a study in which dust samples were collected from the living rooms of 182 single family dwellings in six cities in Japan. The prevalence of SBS, asthma, atopic dermatitis, allergic rhinitis and conjunctivitis was 6.5%, 4.7%, 10.3%, 7.6% and 14.9%, respectively. Significant associations between the medical treatment of asthma and floor bis (2-ethylhexyl) adipate (DEHA) and multi-surface di-n-butyl phthalate (DnBP), dermatitis and floor BBzP and DEHA, conjunctivitis and floor Bis(2-ethylhexyl) phthalate (DEHP) were obtained after adjustment.

Office buildings normally have very low concentrations of **mites**, because they do not provide appropriate conditions for their growth. **Mites** are, however, relatively abundant in household dust. They can be destroyed by keeping absolute humidity below 7 g/kg of air (about 45%) during the winter time (ECA 1989). **Airborne house dust** frequently causes allergic symptoms. However, house dust may also be problematic for healthy subjects without hypersensitivity reactions, as presented by Mølhave et al. (2000). This Danish Office Dust Experiment (Mølhave et al. 2000) investigated the response of 24 healthy non-sensitive adult subjects to the exposure to **normal office dust** in the air. The responses were both subjective sensory reactions and other neurogenic effects even at exposure levels within the range found in normal buildings. Some of the effects appeared acutely and decreased through adaptation, while others increased during prolonged exposure and remained for more than 17 h after the exposure had ended. The threshold level for the dose-response relationships was below 140 $\mu g/m^3$.

BOX 3.10 Dose-response relationship

The dose-response relationship, or exposure-response relationship, describes the change in effect on an organism caused by differing levels of exposure (or doses) to a stressor (usually chemical) after a certain exposure time, or to a food (Crump et al. 1976).

3.6   Association Between Potential Health Outcomes and Psychosocial Health Risk Factors in Built Environments

The category of psychosocial, personal and other risk factors for SBS includes gender, individual characteristics, health condition, stress, feelings of loneliness and helplessness, working position, social status, and others.

> **Gender, working position, and health characteristics** are important health determinants. They cannot be controlled by individuals (WHO 2017a) but have to be carefully considered in the design process.

Stenberg et al. (1994) made a screening questionnaire study of 4,943 office workers and a case-referent study of SBS in 464 subjects. In the study, **females** reported SBS more often than males did. The same conclusions were found in the studies by Sun et al. (2013) in a dormitory environment in Tianjin, China (2006–2007) and in a study by Engvall et al. (2000) in multi-family buildings in Stockholm. Additionally, the influence and importance of **gender** on the prevalence of the SBS symptoms were investigated on 590 employees of three office buildings in Norway (Lenvik 1993). The results showed that a greater percentage of **females** than males reported having the SBS symptoms.

Women are often employed under less favourable working conditions than men, as was confirmed in the study by Bullinger et al. (1999). Questionnaire results from 2,517 female employees in Germany (as compared to 2,079 male employees) showed that women report higher scores in sensory irritation, a higher bodily complaint rate, and a more negative evaluation of the indoor climate. In addition, most psychosocial variables showed less favourable scores for women as compared to men.

The relative influence of **gender, atopy, smoking habits**, and **age** on reported SBS symptoms among office workers was investigated through questionnaire studies among 1,293 employees in 10 nonindustrial buildings (Lenvik 1993). The occurrence of atopy among the office workers was not found to be different from that of the general population. The prevalence of symptoms was higher among atopic individuals than among nonatopics and higher among females than among males. While gender was found to be important for some symptoms, atopy was important for all of them. The results indicated interrelations between smoking and atopy, with the enhanced prevalence of some symptoms. The age of the persons was also included in the analyses. Different ways of grouping age indicated different trends in associations between age and the prevalence of symptoms, but the study did not show any unambiguous associations between the age and the prevalence of symptoms. The same conclusion was made in the literature review by

Norbäck (2009), showing that there was no consistent association between **age** and SBS.

Symptoms are generally more common and more problematic in the **stressed**, the **unloved**, and in **individuals who feel powerless** to change their situation. There is a strong association between **lack of control** of the office environment and symptoms and an association between lower social status and the SBS symptoms (Burge 2004). Norlen and Andersson (1993) showed that residents in **single-family** houses reported less SBS than those in **multifamily** houses, although measurements suggest a less favourable indoor environment in single-family houses.

> **Occupational stress** has been shown to have a detrimental effect on the health and wellbeing of employees, as well as a negative impact on workplace productivity and profits (Bickford 2005).

Some researchers (Morris and Hawkins 1987; Hedge et al. 1987) have investigated the possible links between SBS symptoms and **occupational stress**. Occupational stress has been found to be correlated with SBS symptoms, but much of the research has been of a cross-sectional nature, and it does not indicate whether stress is an active element or an outcome (Crawford and Bolas 1996). However, Ooi and Goh (1997) examined the role of **work-related psychosocial stress** among 2160 subjects in 67 offices in the aetiology of SBS. Ooi and Goh (1997) found an incremental trend in the prevalence of SBS among office workers who reported high levels of **physical** and **mental stress**, and a decreasing climate of **co-operation**.

Lu et al. (2007) investigated whether SBS complaints and indoor air pollution for 389 office workers in 87 government offices of eight high-rise buildings in Taipei, Taiwan are associated with oxidative stress. **Oxidative stress** was indicated by urinary 8-hydroxydeoxyguanosine (8-OHdG). The results showed that urinary 8-OHdG had significant associations with VOC and CO_2 in offices, and with urinary cotinine levels. The mean urinary 8-OHdG level was also significantly higher in participants with the SBS symptoms than in those without such complaints. The mean 8-OHdG increased as the number of SBS symptoms increased. This study indicated that the 8-OHdG level was closely associated with the SBS complaints after controlling the air pollution and smoking.

3.7 Association Between Potential Health Outcomes and Other Factors in Built Environments

In previous sections of this chapter, specific health risk factors in built environments were defined, presenting quite well-researched topics. However, in the first chapter, it was described that numerous health determinants impact built environments; many of them are poorly researched. Additionally, due to the specific characteristics of risk factors, some of the measurement techniques and analyses remain partly or even non-defined.

Other health risk factors in built environments for which health outcomes were proved by studies are: **location, building characteristics, ownership, presence of insecticides, geopathogenic zones** and **geopathic stress**, etc.

Wang et al. (2013) performed a study in domestic environments in Chongqing, China and confirmed that **living near a main road or highway, redecoration, and new furniture** were risk factors for perceptions of odours and sensations of humid air and dry air. The presence of **cockroaches, rats, and mosquitoes/flies, use of mosquito-repellent incense** and other incenses were all risk factors. The analyses of 609 multi-family buildings with 14,235 dwellings in Stockholm (Engvall et al. 2000) showed that subjects **owning buildings** reported less SBS, but the relationship between **ownership** and **building age** was strong. According to the model, 5% of all buildings built before 1961, 13% of those built in 1976–1984, and 15% of those built in 1985–1990 would have significantly more SBS than expected. Another issue that has to be investigated in relation to SBS is **geopathogenic zones** and **geopathic stress**.

BOX 3.11 Geopathic stress

The word "geopathic" is derived from two Greek words: *geo*, meaning "of the earth" and *pathos*, meaning "suffering" or "disease". Geopathic stress can undermine both the body's subtle energy system (the etheric body, chakras and meridians) and the body's electrical system (brain, heart and muscles), thus delaying healing and recovery. Interest in geopathic stress first arose in Germany in the 1920s (Freshwater 1997).

Augner et al. (2010) evaluated whether two different locations in the same room as tested by dowsers ("geopathic stress zone" versus "more neutral zone") would show significant short-term effects on work performance and well-being. The authors performed a blinded, randomized, short-term laboratory experiment (N = 26 persons, aged 20–57). Analysis of variance revealed a trend (p = 0.07) and showed significantly **poorer well-being under the geopathic stress zone** condition compared to a **more neutral zone** (p = 0.01). No location-dependent effects on performance during the reactive stress tolerance test were seen.

References

Abdel-Hamid, M. A., Hakim, S. A., Elokda, E. E., & Mostafa, N. S. (2013). Prevalence and risk factors of sick building syndrome among office workers. *The Journal of The Egyptian Public Health Association 88*(2), 109–114. https://doi.org/10.1097/01.EPX.0000431629.28378.c0.

Adams, R. I., Bhangar, S., Dannemiller, K. C., Eisen, J. A., Fierer, N., Gilbert, J. A., et al. (2016). Ten questions concerning the microbiomes of buildings. *Building and Environment 109*, 224–234. https://doi.org/10.1016/j.buildenv.2016.09.001.

Al-Hunaiti, A., Arar, S., Täubel, M., Wraith, D., Maragkidou, A., Hyvärinen, A., et al. (2017) Floor dust bacteria and fungi and their coexistence with PAHs in Jordanian indoor environments. *Science of the Total Environment 601*, 940–945. https://doi.org/10.1016/j. scitotenv.2017.05.211.

Alexander, D. D., Bailey, W. H., Perez, V., Mitchell, M.E., & Su, S. (2013). Air ions and respiratory function outcomes: A comprehensive review. *Journal of Negative Results in Biomedicine 12*(14), 1–16. https://doi.org/10.1186/1477-5751-12-14.

Amin, N. D. M., Akasah, Z.A., & Razzaly, W. (2015). Architectural evaluation of thermal comfort: Sick building syndrome symptoms in engineering education laboratories. *Procedia— Social and Behavioral Sciences 204*, 19–28. Retrieved November 10, 2018, from http://www. sciencedirect.com/science/article/pii/S1877042815047539.

Ammann, H. M. (1988). Microbial volatile organic compounds. In J. M. Macher (Ed.) *Bioaerosols: Assessment and Control, ACGIH, Cincinnati, UH, 1988* (pp. 26-1–26-17).

Andersen, I., Lundqvist, G. R., Jensen, P. L., & Proctor, D. F. (1974). Human response to 78-hour exposure to dry air. *Archives of Environmental Health: An International Journal 29*(6), 319–324.

Apte, M. G., Fisk, W. J., & Daisey, J. M. (2000). Associations between indoor CO_2 concentrations and sick building syndrome symptoms in U.S. Office buildings: An analysis of the 1994–1996 BASE study data. *Indoor Air 10*, 246–257. https://doi.org/10.1034/j.1600-0668.2000. 010004246.x.

Araki, A., Kawai, T., Eitaki, Y., Kanazawa, A., Morimoto K., Nakayama, K., et al. (2010). Relationship between selected indoor volatile organic compounds, so-called microbial VOC, and the prevalence of mucous membrane symptoms in single family homes. *Science of the Total Environment 408*(10), 2208–2215. https://doi.org/10.1016/j.scitotenv.2010.02.012.

ARB. (2012). Air Resources Board, Indoor air quality guideline. Retrieved November 10, 2018, from http://www.arb.ca.gov/research/indoor/formaldGL08-04.pdf.

ASHRAE Standard 62.1. (2004). Ventilation for acceptable indoor air quality, American Society of Heating, Refrigerating and Air Conditioning Engineers, Atlanta.

Augner, C., Hacker, G. W., & Jekel, I. (2010). Geopathic stress zones: Short-term effects on work performance and well-being? *The Journal of Alternative and Complementary Medicine 16*(6), 657–661. Retrieved December 6, 2018, from https://www.ncbi.nlm.nih.gov/pubmed/20569033 , https://doi.org/10.1089/acm.2009.0499.

Aydogan, A., & Montoya, L. D. (2011) Formaldehyde removal by common indoor plant species and various growing media. *Atmospheric Environment 45*(16), 2675–2682. Retrieved November 10, 2018, from https://www.sciencedirect.com/science/article/pii/ S1352231011002263, https://doi.org/10.1016/j.chemosphere.2018.01.078.

Awbi, H. B. (2003). *Ventilation of buildings* (2nd ed.). New York: Taylor & Francis.

Bakó-Biró, Z., Clements-Croomea, D. J., Kochhara, N., Awbia, H. B., & Williams, M. J. (2007). Ventilation rates in schools and learning performance. In *Finnish Association of HVAC Societies. Proceedings of the 9th REHVA World Congress: Clima 2007 wellbeing indoors; Helsinki, 10–14 June 2007*. Helsinki: Finnish Association of HVAC Societies.

Barna, E., & Bánhidi, L. (2012). Combined effect of two local discomfort parameters studied with a thermal manikin and human subjects. *Energy and Buildings 51*, 234–241. https://doi.org/10. 1016/j.enbuild.2012.05.015.

Beauchemin, K. M., & Hays, P. (1996). Sunny hospital rooms expedite recovery from severe and refractory depressions. *Journal of Affective Disorders, 40*(1–2), 49–51.

Benedetti, F., Colombo, C., Barbini, B., Campori, E., & Smeraldi, E. (2001). Morning sunlight reduces length of hospitalization in bipolar depression. *Journal of Affective Disorders 62*(3), 221–223. https://doi.org/10.1016/S0165-0327(00)00149-X.

Bickford, M. (2005). Stress in the workplace: A general overview of the causes, the effects, and the solutions. Canadian Mental Health Association Newfoundland and Labrador Division.

Biology online. (2017). Bacteria. Retrieved November 11, 2018, from http://www.biology-online. org/dictionary/Bacteria.

Blondel, A., & Plaisance, H. (2011). Screening of formaldehyde indoor sources and quantification of their emission using a passive sampler. *Building and Environment 46*(6), 1284–1291. https://doi.org/10.1016/j.buildenv.2010.12.011.

Bornehag, C. G., Sundell, J, Weschler, C. J., Sigsgaard, T., Lundgren, B,, Hasselgren, M., et al. (2004). The association between asthma and allergic symptoms in children and phthalates in house dust: A nested case–control study. *Environmental Health Perspectives 112,* 1393–1397. https://doi.org/10.1289/ehp.7187.

Bowers, B., Flory, R., Ametepe, J., Staley, L., Patrick, A., & Carrington, H. (2018). Controlled trial evaluation of exposure duration to negative air ions for the treatment of seasonal affective disorder. *Psychiatry Research 259,* 7–14. http://dx.doi.org/10.1016/j.psychres.2017.08.040.

Bullinger, M., Morfeld, M., von Mackensen, S., & Brasche, S. (1999). The sick-building-syndrome—do women suffer more? *Zentralblatt für Hygiene und Umweltmedizin 202*(2–4), 235–241. http://dx.doi.org/10.1016/S0934-8859(99)80025-X.

Burge, P. S., Jones, P., & Robertson, A. S. (1990). Sick building syndrome; environmental comparisons of sick and healthy buildings. *Indoor Air 1,* 479–83.

Burge, P. S. (2004). Sick building syndrome. *Occupational and Environmental Medicine 61,* 185–190. http://dx.doi.org/10.1136/oem.2003.008813.

Butala, V., & Novak, P. (1999). Energy consumption and potential energy savings in old school buildings. *Energy and Buildings, 29*(3), 241–246. https://doi.org/10.1016/S0378-7788(98)00062-0.

CAN/CSA-Z1002-12. (2017). Occupational health and safety—Hazard identification and elimination and risk assessment and control.

Carrer, P., Wargocki, P., Fanetti, A., Bischof, W., Fernandes, E. D. O., Hartmann, T., et al. (2015) What does the scientific literature tell us about the ventilation–health relationship in public and residential buildings? *Building and Environment 94*(1), 273–286. Retrieved November 10, 2018, from http://www.sciencedirect.com/science/article/pii/S0360132315300925, https://doi.org/10.1016/j.buildenv.2015.08.011.

CCOHS. (2011). Canadian centre for occupational health and safety. Environmental tobacco smoke (ETS): General information and health effects. Retrieved November 10, 2018, from http://www.ccohs.ca/oshanswers/psychosocial/ets_health.html.

CDC. (2009). Centers for disease control and prevention. Health risk appraisals. Retrieved November 10, 2018, from https://www.cdc.gov/workplacehealthpromotion/tools-resources/workplace-health/assessment-tools.html.

CDC. (2013). Centers for Disease Control and Prevention. Indoor environmental quality. Retrieved November 10, 2017, from http://www.cdc.gov/niosh/topics/indoorenv/chemicalsodors.html.

Chauhan, R. P., Kant, K., Sharma, S. K., & Chakarvarti, S. K. (2003). Measurement of alpha radioactive air pollutants in fly ash brick dwellings. *Radiation Measurements 36*(1–6), 533–536. Retrieved November 10, 2018, from http://www.sciencedirect.com/science/article/pii/S1350448703001963, http://dx.doi.org/10.1016/S1350-4487(03)00196-3.

Choi, J. H., Beltran, L. O., & Kim, H. S. (2012). Impacts of indoor daylight environments on patient average length of stay (ALOS) in a healthcare facility. *Building and Environment 50,* 65–75. http://dx.doi.org/10.1016/j.buildenv.2011.10.010.

Choi, H., Schmidbauer, N., & Bornehag, C. G. (2017). Volatile organic compounds of possible microbial origin and their risks on childhood asthma and allergies within damp homes. *Environment International, 98,* 143–151. https://doi.org/10.1016/j.envint.2016.10.028.

Clark, L. A., & Watson, D. J. (1988). Mood and the mundane: Relations between daily life events and self-reported mood. *Journal of Personality and Social Psychology, 54*(2), 296–308. https://doi.org/10.1037/0022-3514.54.2.296.

Cohen, A., Janssen, S., & Solomon, G. (2007). Hidden hazards of air fresheners. Natural Resources Defense Council. Clearing the Air, NRDC Issue Paper 2007, pp. 1–16. Retrieved November 10, 2018, from https://www.nrdc.org/health/home/airfresheners/airfresheners.pdf.

Collins. (2017a). Collins English Dictionary. Definition of 'health risk'. Retrieved November 10, 2018, from https://www.collinsdictionary.com/dictionary/english/health-risk.

Collins. (2017b). Collins English Dictionary. Definition of 'health hazard'. Retrieved November 10, 2018, from, https://www.collinsdictionary.com/dictionary/english/health-hazard.

Commission Directive. (1999). Commission Directive 1999/77/EC of 26 July 1999 adapting to technical progress for the sixth time Annex I to Council Directive 76/769/EEC on the approximation of the laws, regulations and administrative provisions of the Member States relating to restrictions on the marketing and use of certain dangerous substances and preparations (asbestos). Retrieved November 10, 2018, from http://eur-lex.europa.eu/LexUriServ/LexUriServ.do?uri=OJ:L:1999:207:0018:0020:EN:PDF.

Costa, M. F., & Brickus, L. S. (2000). Effects of ventilation systems on prevalence of symptoms associated with sick buildings in Brazilian commercial establishments. *Archives of Environmental Health, 55,* 279–283. https://doi.org/10.1080/00039890009603419.

Crawford, J. O., & Bolas, S. M. (1996). Sick building syndrome, work factors and occupational stress. *Scandinavian Journal of Work, Environment & Health, 22*(4), 243–250. https://doi.org/10.5271/sjweh.138.

Crook, B., & Burton, N. C. (2010). Indoor moulds, sick building syndrome and building related illness. *Fungal Biology Reviews, 24*(3–4), 106–113. https://doi.org/10.1016/j.fbr.2010.05.001.

Crump, K. S., Hoel, D. G., Langley, C. H., & Peto, R. (1976). Fundamental carcinogenic processes and their implications for low dose risk assessment. *Cancer Research 36*(9 Part1), 2973–2979.

Dovjak, M., & Kristl, Ž. (2009). Development of the Leonardo da Vinci accessible world for all respecting differences—AWARD project. *International Journal of Sanitary Engineering Research, 2*(3), 35–49.

Dovjak, M., & Kristl, Ž. (2011). Health concerns of PVC materials in the built environment. *International Journal of Sanitary Engineering Research, 5*(1), 4–26.

Dovjak, M., Kukec, A. (2014). Prevention and control of sick building syndrome (SBS). Part 2, Design of a preventive and control strategy to lower the occurrence of SBS. *International Journal of Sanitary Engineering Research 8*(1), 41–55.

Easton, V. J., & McColl, J. H. (1997). Statistics Glossary v1.1. Retrieved December 6, 2018, from, http://www.stats.gla.ac.uk/steps/glossary/.

EC European Commission. (2012). Recommendation from the Scientific Committee on Occupational Exposure. Retrieved November 10, 2018, from, http://ec.europa.eu/social/BlobServlet?docId=7722&langId=en.

ECA European Concerted Action. (1989). Indoor air quality & its impact on man. COST Project 613. Environment and Quality of Life. Report No. 4. Sick Building Syndrome, A Practical Guide. Commission of the European Communities. Directorate General for Science, Research and Development. Joint Research Centre—Institute for the Environment. Luxembourg: Office for Publications of the European Communities. Retrieved November 10, 2018, from http://www.buildingecology.com/publications/ECA_Report4.pdf.

EN 15251. (2007). Indoor environmental input parameters for design and assessment of energy performance of buildings addressing indoor air quality, thermal environment, lighting and acoustics.

Engvall, K., Norrby, C., Bandel, J., Hult, M., & Norbäck, D. (2000). Development of a multiple regression model to identify multi-family residential buildings with a high prevalence of sick building syndrome (SBS). *Indoor Air, 10,* 101–110. https://doi.org/10.1034/j.1600-0668.2000.010002101.x.

EPA. (2012). Environmental Protection Agency. Biological contaminants. Retrieved November 10, 2018, from http://www.epa.gov/iaq/biologic.html.

EPA. (2016). United States environmental protection agency. Risk assessment. Human Health Risk Assessment. Retrieved November 10, 2018, from https://www.epa.gov/risk/human-health-risk-assessment.

EPA. (2017a). Health risk of radon. Retrieved December 6, 2018, from https://www.epa.gov/radon/health-risk-radon.

EPA. (2017b). Indoor Air Quality (IAQ) Volatile organic compounds' impact on indoor air quality. Retrieved November 10, 2018, from https://www.epa.gov/indoor-air-quality-iaq/volatile-organic-compounds-impact-indoor-air-quality.

Erdmann, C. A., Steiner, K. C., & Apte, M. G. (2002). Indoor carbon dioxide concentrations and sick building syndrome symptoms. In *The Base Study Revisited: Analyses of the 100 Building Dataset Proceedings: Indoor Air 2002*, (pp. 443–448).

Erklavec, U., Dovjak, M., Golja, A., & Kukec, A. (2017). Indoor air pollution and health effects: Systematic review. In *21st International Eco-Conference and 12th Eco-Conference on Environmental Protection of Urban and Suburban Settlements*, Novi Sad, Serbia, 27th–29th September 2017 (pp. 39–47).

Eriksson, N. M., & Stenberg, B. G. T. (2006). Baseline prevalence of symptoms related to indoor environment. *Scandinavian Journal of Public Health, 34*, 387–396. https://doi.org/10.1080/14034940500228281.

Freshwater, D. (1997). Geopathic stress. *Complementary Therapies in Nursing and Midwifery, 3* (6), 160–162. Retrieved November 10, 2017, from http://www.sciencedirect.com/science/article/pii/S1353611705810030, https://doi.org/10.1016/S1353-6117(05)81003-0.

Fu, X. (2016). Indoor microbial volatile organic compound (MVOC) levels and associations with respiratory health, sick building syndrome (SBS), and allergy fungi and mycotoxins risk assessment and management. In *Environmental Mycology in Public Health*, (pp. 387–395). Retrieved November 10, 2018, from http://www.sciencedirect.com/science/article/pii/B9780124114715000223, https://doi.org/10.1016/B978-0-12-411471-5.00022-3.

Goodman, N. B., Steinemann, A., Wheeler, A. J., Paevere, P. J., Cheng, M., & Browna, S. K. (2017). Volatile organic compounds within indoor environments in Australia. *Building and Environment, 122*, 116–125. https://doi.org/10.1016/j.buildenv.2017.05.033.

Gottesfeld, P. (2015). Time to ban lead in industrial paints and coatings. *Front Public Health. 3*, 144. Retrieved November 10, 2018, from https://www.ncbi.nlm.nih.gov/pmc/articles/PMC4434842/, https://doi.org/10.3389/fpubh.2015.00144.

Hathaway, W. E., Hargreaves, J. A., Thomson, G. W., & Novintsky, D. (1992). A summary of light related studies. A study into the effects of light on children of elementary school age. A Case of Daylight Robbery. *IRC Internal Report 659*, 11–27. Retrieved November 10, 2017, from http://www.naturallighting.com/cart/store.php?sc_page=62.

Hedge, A., Sterling, E. M., Collett, C. W., & Mueller B (1987) Indoor air quality investigation as a psychological stressor. In *Proceedings of the 4th Intern. Conf. on Indoor Air Quality and Climate, Indoor Air '87, Berlin (West) 17–21 August 1987* (vol. 2, pp. 552–556). Berlin: Inst. fur Wasser-, Boden- und Lufthygiene.

Hedge, A., & Erickson, W. A. (1998). Sick building syndrome and office ergonomics: A targeted work environment analysis. Human Factors Laboratory, Department of Design & Environmental Analysis, College of Human Ecology, Cornell University, Technology & Engineering.

Heerwagen, J. H. (1986). The role of nature in the view from the window. In S. Zdepski, & V. McCluney (Eds.) *International Daylighting Conference Proceedings II*, November 4–7, 1986. International Daylighting Organizing Committee, Long Beach, CA, pp. 430–437.

Hendrick, D. J., & Lane, D. J. (1977). Occupational forrnalin asthma. *British Journal of Industrial Medicine, 34*, 11–18.

Hess-Kosa, K. (2002). *Indoor air quality: The latest sampling and analytical methods*, 2nd edn. CRC Press.

Heudorf, U., Mersch-Sundermann, V., & Angerer, J. (2007). Phthalates: Toxicology and exposure. *International Journal of Hygiene and Environmental Health, 210*(5), 623–634. https://doi.org/10.1016/j.ijheh.2007.07.011.

Hodgson, M. J., Permar, E., Squire, G., Cagney, W., Allen, A., & Parkinson, D. K. (1987). Vibrations as a cause of "tight-building syndrome" symptoms. *Ibid 2*, 449–453.

Hodgson, M. (2002). Indoor environmental exposures and symptoms. *Environmental health perspectives, 110*, 663–667. https://doi.org/10.1289/ehp.02110s4663.

HSA. (2017). Health and safety authority. healthy, safe and productive lives. Hazard and risk. Retrieved November 10, 2017, from http://www.hsa.ie/eng/Topics/Hazards/.

IARC. (2002). International agency for research on cancer. Monographs on the evaluation of carcinogenic risks to humans. In *Man-Made Vitrous Fibres 2002* (vol. 81). IARC Press, Lyon.

ILO. (2011). International Labour Organization. Indoor air ionization. Retrieved November 10, 2018, from http://www.ilo.org/oshenc/part-vi/indoor-environmental-control/item/261-indoor-air-ionization.

ISO 7726. (1998). Ergonomics of the thermal environment—Instruments for measuring physical quantities.

Jaakkola, J. J. K., Heinonen, O. P., & Seppänen, O. (1989). Sick building syndrome, sensation of dryness and thermal comfort in relation to room temperature in an office building: Need for individual control of temperature. *Environment International, 15,* 163–168. https://doi.org/10.1016/0160-4120(89)90022-6.

Jaakkola, J. J., Oie, L., Nafstad, P., Botten, G., Samuelsen, S. O., & Magnus, P. (1999). Interior surface materials in the home and development of bronchial obstruction in young children in Oslo, Norway. *American Journal of Public Health, 89*(2), 188–192. https://doi.org/10.2105/AJPH.89.2.188.

Jaakkola, J. J. K., & Knight, T. L. (2008). The role of exposure to phthalates from Polyvinyl Chloride products in the development of asthma and allergies: A systematic review and meta-analysis. *Environmental Health Perspectives, 116*(7), 845–853. https://doi.org/10.1289/ehp.10846.

Jokl, M. V. (1989). *Microenvironment, the theory and practice of indoor climate.* Illinois: Charles C Thomas Pub Ltd.

Kameda, T., Takahashi, K., Kim, R., Jiang, Y., Movahed, M., Park, E.-K., et al. (2014). *Bull World Health Organ 92*(11), 790–797. Retrieved November 10, 2017, from https://www.ncbi.nlm.nih.gov/pmc/articles/PMC4221761/, http://dx.doi.org/10.2471/BLT.13.132118.

Kishi, R., Araki, A., Saitoh, I., Shibata, E., Morimoto, K., Nakayama, K., et al. (2012). Phthalate in house dust and its relation to sick building syndrome and allergic symptoms. In *30th International Congress on Occupational Health organized in Cancun from March 18th to March 23rd, 2012.* Mexico: ICOH.

Korpi, A., Järnberg, J., & Pasanen, A. L. (2009). Microbial volatile organic compounds. *Critical Reviews in Toxicology, 39*(2), 139–193. https://doi.org/10.1080/10408440802291497.

Kukec, A., Dovjak, M. (2014). Prevention and control of sick building syndrome (SBS). Part 1, Identification of risk factors. *International Journal of Sanitary Engineering Research 8*(1), 16–40.

Lantz, P. M., Mendez, D., & Philbert, M. (2013). Radon, smoking, and lung cancer: The need to refocus radon control policy. *American Journal of Public Health 103*(3), 443–447. Retrieved December 6, 2018, from https://www.ncbi.nlm.nih.gov/pmc/articles/PMC3673501/, http://dx.doi.org/10.2105/AJPH.2012.300926.

Lenvik, K. (1993). Smoking habits, atopy, and prevalence of sick building syndrome symptoms among office workers in Norway. *Environment International, 19*(4), 333–340. https://doi.org/10.1016/0160-4120(93)90125-2.

Li, C. S., Hsu, C. W., & Lu, C. H. (1997). Dampness and respiratory symptoms among workers in day-care centers in a subtropical climate. *Archives of Environmental Health, 52,* 68–71. https://doi.org/10.1080/00039899709603803.

Lim, F. L., Hashim, Z., Md Said, S., Than, L. T., Hashim, J. H., & Norbäck, D. (2015). Sick building syndrome (SBS) among office workers in a Malaysian university-associations with atopy, fractional exhaled nitric oxide (FeNO) and the office environment. *Science of the Total Environment, 1*(536), 353–361. https://doi.org/10.1016/j.scitotenv.2015.06.137.

Liu, Y.-J., Mu, Y.-J., Zhu, Y.-G., Ding, H., & Arens, N. C. (2007). Which ornamental plant species effectively remove benzene from indoor air? *Atmospheric Environment 41*(3), 650–654. Retrieved November 10, 2018, from http://www.sciencedirect.com/science/article/pii/S1352231006008077, http://dx.doi.org/10.1016/j.atmosenv.2006.08.001.

Logue, J. M., McKone, T. E., Sherman, M. H., & Singer, B. C. (2011). Hazard assessment of chemical air contaminants measured in residences. *Indoor Air, 21*(2), 92–109. https://doi.org/10.1111/j.1600-0668.2010.00683.x.

Lu, C. Y., Ma, Y. C., Lin, J. M., Li, C. Y., Lin, R. S., & Sung, F. C. (2007). Oxidative stress associated with indoor air pollution and sick building syndrome-related symptoms among office workers in Taiwan. *Inhalation Toxicology, 19*(1), 57–65. https://doi.org/10.1080/08958370600985859.

Madigan, M., & Martinko, J. (Eds.). (2005). *Brock biology of microorganisms* (11th ed.). Upper Saddle River, NJ: Prentice Hall.

Markussen, S., & Røed, K. (2014). Daylight and absenteeism—Evidence from Norway. *Economics & Human Biology, 16,* 73–80. https://doi.org/10.1016/j.ehb.2014.01.002.

Marsili, D., Terracini, B., Santana, V. S., Ramos-Bonilla, J. P., Pasetto, R., Mazzeo, A., et al. (2016). Prevention of asbestos-related disease in countries currently using asbestos. *International Journal of Environmental Research and Public Health 13*(5), 494. Retrieved November 10, 2018, from https://www.ncbi.nlm.nih.gov/pmc/articles/PMC4881119/, http://dx.doi.org/10.3390/ijerph13050494.

Mizoue, T., Reijula, K., & Andersson, K. (2001). Environmental tobacco smoke exposure and overtime work as risk factors for sick building syndrome in Japan. *American Journal of Epidemiology, 154*(9), 803–808. https://doi.org/10.1093/aje/154.9.803.

Mølhave, L., Kjærgaard, S. K., & Attermann, J. (2000). Sensory and other neurogenic effects of exposures to airborne office dust. *Atmospheric Environment, 34*(28), 4755–4766. https://doi.org/10.1016/S1352-2310(00)00266-1.

Mølhave, L. (2003). Organic compounds as indicators of air pollution. *Indoor Air, 13*(6), 12–19. https://doi.org/10.1034/j.1600-0668.13.s.6.2.x.

Morris, L., Hawkins, L. (1987). The role of stress in the sick building syndrome. In *Proceedings of the 4th International Conference on Indoor Air Quality and Climate, Indoor Air '87, Berlin (West), 17–21 August 1987* (vol. 2, pp. 566–571). Berlin: Inst. fur Wasser, Boden und Lufthygiene.

Nakaoka, H., Todaka, E., Seto, H., Saito, I., Hanazato, M., Watanabe, M., et al. (2014). Correlating the symptoms of sick-building syndrome to indoor VOCs concentration levels and odour. *Indoor and Built Environment, 23*(6), 804–813. https://doi.org/10.1177/1420326X13500975.

NDA. (2014). National Disability Authority. What is universal design. Retrieved November 10, 2018, from http://universaldesign.ie/What-is-Universal-Design/.

Nexo, E., Skov, P. G., & Gravesen, S. (1983). Extreme fatique and malaise syndrome caused by badly-cleaned wall-to-wall carpets? *Ecology of Disease, 2,* 415–418.

Nicklas, M. H., & Bailey, G. B. (1997). Analysis of the performance of students in daylight schools. In *Proceedings of the 1997 Annual Conference, ASES* (pp. 1–5). Colorado: American Solar Energy Society.

Nielsen, O. (1987). Man-made mineral fibers in the indoor climate caused by ceilings of man-made mineral wool. In B. Seifert, H. Esdorn, M. Fisher, H. Riiden, & J. Wegner (Eds.) *Proceedings of the 4th International Conference on Indoor Air Quality and Climate Indoor Air '87*, (vol. 1, pp. 580–583). Berlin: Institute for Water, Soil and Air Hygiene.

NIH. (2017). National heart, lung, and blood institute. Risk factors. Retrieved November 10, 2018, from https://www.nhlbi.nih.gov/health/health-topics/topics/obe/risks.

NIOSH. (1976). National Institute for Occupational Safety and Health. Criteria for a recommended standard, occupational exposure to carbon dioxide. Retrieved November 10, 2018, from http://www.cdc.gov/niosh/docs/1970/76-194.html.

NIPH. (2009). Nacionalni inštitut za varovanje zdravja RS, Osvežilci zraka. Retrieved November 10, 2018, from http://www.ivz.si/Mp.aspx?ni=78&pi=6&_6_id=286&_6_PageIndex=0&_6_groupId=-2&_6_newsCategory=IVZ+kategorija&_6_action=ShowNewsFull&pl=78-6.0.

Norbäck, D. (2009). An update on sick building syndrome: Personal risk factors for sick building syndrome. In *Medscape, 2009*. Retrieved November 10, 2018, from http://www.medscape.org/viewarticle/701739_7.

Norbäck, D., Hashim, J. H., Hashim, Z., & Ali, F. (2017). Volatile organic compounds (VOC), formaldehyde and nitrogen dioxide (NO_2) in schools in Johor Bahru, Malaysia: Associations with rhinitis, ocular, throat and dermal symptoms, headache and fatigue. *Science of the Total Environment, 592,* 153–160. https://doi.org/10.1016/j.scitotenv.2017.02.215.

Nordström, K., Norbäck, D., & Akselsson, R. (1994). Effect of air humidification on the sick building syndrome and perceived indoor air quality in hospitals: A four month longitudinal study. *Occupational and Environmental Medicine 51*(10), 683–688. Retrieved November 10, 2018, from https://www.ncbi.nlm.nih.gov/pmc/articles/PMC1128077/.

Norhidayah, A., Chia-Kuang, Lee, Azhar, M. K., & Nurulwahida, S. (2013). Indoor air quality and sick building syndrome in three selected buildings. *Procedia Engineering, 53,* 93–98. https://doi.org/10.1016/j.proeng.2013.02.014.

Norlen, U., Andersson, K. (1993). An indoor climate survey of the Swedish housing stock (the ELIB study). In *Proceedings of Indoor Air '93, 6th International Conference on Indoor Air Quality and Climate, Helsinki* (vol. 1, pp. 743–748).

OJ RS. (2002). OJ RS No. 42/2002, 105/2002: Rules on the ventilation and air-conditioning of buildings.

Ooi, P. L., & Goh, K. T. (1997). Sick building syndrome: An emerging stress-related disorder? *International Journal of Epidemiology, 26*(6), 1243–1249. https://doi.org/10.1093/ije/26.6.1243.

OSHA. (2017). Occupational Safety and Health Administration. Health Hazard Definitions Regulations (Standards - 29 CFR)—Table of Contents. Retrieved November 10, 2018, from https://www.osha.gov/pls/oshaweb/owadisp.show_document?p_table=STANDARDS&p_id=10371.

Pantoja, L. D. M., Nascimento, R. F., & Nunes, A. B. A. N. (2016). Investigation of fungal volatile organic compounds in hospital air. *Atmospheric Pollution Research, 7*(4), 659–663. https://doi.org/10.1016/j.apr.2016.02.011.

Park, S., Seo, J., & Kim, J. T. (2015). A study on the application of sorptive building materials to reduce the concentration and volume of contaminants inhaled by occupants in office areas. *Energy and Buildings 98,* 10–18. Retrieved November 10, 2018, from http://www.sciencedirect.com/science/article/pii/S0378778815000195, http://dx.doi.org/10.1016/j.enbuild.2014.12.056.

Petrović, E. K. (2017). 8-New and less recognized risks with building materials: Volatile organic compounds, replacement chemicals, and nanoparticles. Materials for a healthy, ecological and sustainable built environment. Principles for evaluation. A volume in Woodhead Publishing Series in Civil and Structural Engineering (pp. 191–202)

Pheasant, S. (1986). *Body space: Anthropometry ergonomics and design.* London: Taylor & Francis.

Pheasant, S. (1987). Review of: "Ergonomics-standards and guidelines for designers" By Stephen Pheasant (London: BSI Standards, 1987). *Ergonomics 31*(8), 1214–1215.

Pheasant, S. (1991). *Ergonomics, work and health* (p. 358). London: MacMillan Press, Houndmills.

Porta, M. (2008). *A dictionary of epidemiology (Sixth Edition).* International Epidemiological Association, Oxford University Press. Retrieved November 10, 2018, from http://irea.ir/files/site1/pages/dictionary.pdf.

Prek, M., & Butala, V. (2012). An enhanced thermal comfort model based on the energy analysis approach. *International Journal of Exergy, 10*(2), 190–208. https://doi.org/10.1504/IJEX.2012.045865.

Redlich, C. A., Sparer, J., & Cullen, M. R. (1997). Sick-building syndrome. *Lancet, 349,* 1013–1016. https://doi.org/10.1016/S0140-6736(96)07220-0.

Reilly, T., & Stevenson, I. C. (1993). An investigation of the effects of negative air ions on responses to submaximal exercise at different times of day. *Journal of Human Ergology, 22*(1), 1–9.

Robbins, C. L. (1986). *Daylighting: Design and analysis* (pp. 4–13). New York: Van Nostrand Reinhold Company.

Robertson, A. S., Burge, P. S., Hedge, A., Wilson, S., & HarrisBass, J. (1988). Relation between passive cigarette smoking exposure and "building sickness". *Thorax, 43J,* 2638.

Safeopedia. (2017). Health Hazard (OSHA). Retrieved November 10, 2018, from https://www. safeopedia.com/definition/4896/health-hazard-osha.

Sahlberg, B., Gunnbjörnsdottir, M., Soon, A., Jogi, R., Gislason, T., Wieslander, G., et al. (2013). Airborne molds and bacteria, microbial volatile organic compounds (MVOC), plasticizers and formaldehyde in dwellings in three North European cities in relation to sick building syndrome (SBS). *Science of the Total Environment, 444,* 433–440. https://doi.org/10.1016/j.scitotenv. 2012.10.114.

Sakai, K., Norbäck, D., Mi, S., Shibata, E., Kamijima, M., Yamada, T., et al. (2004). A comparison of indoor air pollutants in Japan and Sweden: Formaldehyde, nitrogen dioxide, and chlorinated volatile organic compounds. *Environmental Research, 94*(1), 75–85. https:// doi.org/10.1016/S0013-9351(03)00140-3.

Salthammer, T., Mentese, S., & Marutzky, R. (2010). Formaldehyde in the Indoor Environment. *Chemical Reviews, 110*(4), 2536–2572. https://doi.org/10.1021/cr800399g.

Schneider, T., Sundell, J., Bischof, W., Bohgard, M., Cherrie, J. W., Clausen, P. A., et al. (2003). Airborne particles in the indoor environment. A European interdisciplinary review of scientific evidence on associations between exposure to particles in buildings and health effects. *Indoor Air, 13,* 38–48. https://doi.org/10.1034/j.1600-0668.2003.02025.x.

Seppänen, O. A., Fisk, W. J., & Mendell, M. J. (1999). Association of ventilation rates and CO_2 concentrations with health and other responses in commercial and industrial buildings. *Indoor Air, 9,* 226–252. https://doi.org/10.1111/j.1600-0668.1999.00003.x.

Seppänen, O., & Fisk, W. J. (2002). Association of ventilation system type with SBS symptoms in office workers. *Indoor air, 12,* 98–112. https://doi.org/10.1034/j.1600-0668.2002.01111.x.

Simmons, L. H., & Richard, J. L. (1997). *Building materials: Dangerous properties of products.* River Street: Wiley.

Stenberg, B., Eriksson, N., Höög, J., Sundell, J., & Wall, S. (1994). The sick building syndrome (SBS) in office workers. A case-referent study of personal, psychosocial and building related risk indicators. *International Journal of Epidemiology, 23,* 1190–1197. https://doi.org/10.1093/ ije/23.6.1190.

Straus, D. C. (2009). Molds, mycotoxins, and sick building syndrome. *Toxicology and Industrial Health, 25*(9–10), 617–635. https://doi.org/10.1177/0748233709348287.

Subedi, B., Sullivan, K. D., & Dhungana, B. (2017). Phthalate and non-phthalate plasticizers in indoor dust from childcare facilities, salons, and homes across the USA. *Environmental Pollution, 230,* 701–708. https://doi.org/10.1016/j.envpol.2017.07.028.

Sulman, F. G. (1980a). The effect of air ionization, electric fields, atmospherics and other electric phenomena on man and animal. Illinois: Thomas.

Sulman, F. G. (1980b). Migraine and headache due to weather and allied causes and its specific treatment. *Upsala Journal of Medical Sciences. Supplement, 31,* 41–44.

Sun, Y., Zhang, Y., Bao, L., Fan, Z., Wang, D., & Sundell, J. (2013). Effects of gender and dormitory environment on sick building syndrome symptoms among college students in Tianjin, China. *Building and Environment, 68,* 134–139. https://doi.org/10.1016/j.buildenv. 2013.06.010.

Szumilas, M. (2010). Explaining odds ratios. *Journal of the Canadian Academy of Child and Adolescent Psychiatry, 19*(3), 227–229.

Šestan, P., Kristl, Ž., & Dovjak, M. (2013). Formaldehyde in the built environment and its potential impact on human health. *Gradbeni Vestnik, 62,* 191–203.

Takigawa, T., Wang, B. L., Sakano, N., Wang, D. H., Ogino, K., & Kishi, R. (2009). A longitudinal study of environmental risk factors for subjective symptoms associated with sick building syndrome in new dwellings. *Science of the Total Environment, 407*(19), 5223–5228. https://doi.org/10.1016/j.scitotenv.2009.06.023.

Takigawa, T., Saijo, Y., Morimoto, K., Nakayama, K., Shibata, E., Tanaka, M., et al. (2012). A longitudinal study of aldehydes and volatile organic compounds associated with subjective symptoms related to sick building syndrome in new dwellings in Japan. *Science of the Total Environment, 417–418,* 61–67. https://doi.org/10.1016/j.scitotenv.2011.12.060.

Teeuw, K. B., Vandenbroucke-Grauls, C. M., & Verhoef, J. (1994). Airborne gram-negative bacteria and endotoxin in sick building syndrome. A study in Dutch governmental office buildings. *Archives of Internal Medicine 154*(20), 2339–2345. http://dx.doi.org/10.1001/archinte.154.20.2339.

Terman, M., Fairhurst, S., Perlman, B., Levitt, J., & McCluney, R. (1986). Daylight deprivation and replenishment: A psychobiological problem with a naturalistic solution. In S. Zdepski, & R. McCluney (Eds.) *International Daylighting Conference Proceedings II, November 4–7, 1986* (pp. 438–443). Long Beach, CA: International Daylighting Organizing Committee.

Tsai, D. H., Lin, J. S., & Chan, C. C. (2012). Office workers' sick building syndrome and indoor carbon dioxide concentrations. *Journal of Occupational and Environmental Hygiene, 9*(5), 345–351. https://doi.org/10.1080/15459624.2012.675291.

UNEP. (2016). Global report on the status of legal limits on lead in paint united nations environment programme 2016. Retrieved November 10, 2018, from https://wedocs.unep.org/bitstream/handle/20.500.11822/11348/Limits-Lead-Paint-2016%20Report-Final.pdf?sequence=1&isAllowed=y.

Valbjorn, O., & Kousgaard, N. (1986). Headache and mucous membrane irritation at home and at work. Report 175. Harsholm: Statens Byggeforsknings Institut (SBI).

Valbjorn, O., & Skov, P. (1987). The Danish Indoor climate study group. Influence of indoor climate on the sick building syndrome prevalence. In *Proceedings of the 4th International Conference on Indoor Air Quality and Climate, Indoor air 1987, Berlin (West) 17–21 August 1987,* (vol. 2, pp. 593–597). Berlin: Inst. fur Wasser, Boden und Lufthygiene.

Wang, S., Ang, H. M., & Tade, M. O. (2007). Volatile organic compounds in indoor environment and photocatalytic oxidation: State of the art. *Environment International, 33,* 694–705. https://doi.org/10.1016/j.envint.2007.02.011.

Wang, J., Li, B., Yang, Q., Yu, W., Wang, W., Norback, D., et al. (2013). Odors and sensations of humidity and dryness in relation to sick building syndrome and home environment in Chongqing, China. *PLoS One, 8*(8), e72385. https://doi.org/10.1371/journal.pone.0072385.

Webb. (2006). Considerations for lighting in the built environment: Non-visual effects of light. Retrieved November 10, 2018, from http://www.livingdaylights.nl/wp-content/uploads/2016/12/Webb-2006.-Considerations-for-lighting-in-the-built-envrionment-Non-visual-effects-of-light..pdf.

WHO. (2004). World Health Organisation. Electromagnetic hypersensitivity. Retrieved November 10, 2018, from http://www.who.int/peh-emf/publications/reports/EHS_Proceedings_June2006.pdf?ua=1.

WHO. (2009a). World Health Organization. Global health risks. Mortality and burden of disease attributable to selected major risks. Retrieved November 10, 2018, from http://www.who.int/healthinfo/global_burden_disease/GlobalHealthRisks_report_full.pdf?ua=1&ua=1.

WHO. (2009b). Night noise guidelines for Europe. Retrieved October 10, 2018, from http://www.euro.who.int/__data/assets/pdf_file/0017/43316/E92845.pdf?ua=1.

WHO. (2009c). World Health Organization. Dampness and mould. Retrieved November 10, 2018, from http://www.euro.who.int/__data/assets/pdf_file/0017/43325/E92645.pdf.

WHO. (2010). Childhood lead poisoning. Retrieved November 10, 2018, from http://www.who.int/ceh/publications/leadguidance.pdf.

WHO. (2013). World Health Organisation. Environment and health. Retrieved November 10, 2018, from http://www.euro.who.int/en/health-topics/environment-and-health/noise.

WHO. (2014). World Health Organisation. Environment and health. Electromagnetic fields (EMF). Retrieved November 10, 2018, from http://www.who.int/peh-emf/about/WhatisEMF/en/index1.html.

WHO. (2017a). Health Impact Assessment (HIA). The determinants of health. Retrieved November 10, 2018, from http://www.who.int/hia/evidence/doh/en/.

WHO. (2017b). Health topics risk factors. Retrieved November 10, 2018, from http://www.who.int/topics/risk_factors/en/.

WHO. (2017c). International programme on chemical safety. Asbestos. Retrieved November 10, 2018, from http://www.who.int/ipcs/assessment/public_health/asbestos/en/.

Wolkoff, P. (1987). Sampling of VOC under conditions of high time resolution. In *Proceedings of the 4th Intern. Conf. on Indoor Air Quality and Climate, Indoor Air '87, Berlin (West), 17–21 August 1987* (vol. 1, pp. 126–129). Berlin: Inst. fur Wasser, Boden und Lufthygiene.

Wonga, S. K. (2009). Sick building syndrome and perceived indoor environmental quality: A survey of apartment buildings in Hong Kong. *Habitat International, 33*(4), 463–471. https://doi.org/10.1016/j.habitatint.2009.03.001.

Xu, Y., Hubal, E. A., Clausen, P. A., & Little, J. C. (2009). Predicting residential exposure to phthalate plasticizer emitted from vinyl flooring: A mechanistic analysis. *Environmental Science and Technology, 43*(7), 2374–2380. https://doi.org/10.1021/es801354f.

Yassi, A., Kjellstrom, T., de Kok, T., & Guidotti, T. (2001). *Basic environmental health*. New York: Oxford University Press Inc.

Yu, B. F., Hu, Z. B., Liu, M., Yang, H. L., Kong, Q. X., & Liu, Y. H. (2009). Review of research on air-conditioning systems and indoor air quality control for human health. *International Journal of Refrigeration, 32*(1), 3–20. https://doi.org/10.1016/j.ijrefrig.2008.05.004.

Yu, C. W. F., & Kim, J. T. (2012). Long-term impact of formaldehyde and VOC emissions from wood-based products on indoor environments and issues with recycled products. *Indoor Built Environment, 21*, 137–149. https://doi.org/10.1177/1420326X11424330.

Zhang, X., Zhao, Z., Nordquist, T., Larsson, L., Sebastian, A., & Norback, D. (2011). A longitudinal study of sick building syndrome among pupils in relation to microbial components in dust in schools in China. *Science of the Total Environment, 409*(24), 5253–5259. https://doi.org/10.1016/j.scitotenv.2011.08.059.

Zhang, X., Sahlberg, B., Wieslander, G., Janson, C., Gislason, T., & Norback, D. (2012). Dampness and moulds in workplace buildings: Associations with incidence and remission of sick building syndrome (SBS) and biomarkers of inflammation in a 10-year follow-up study. *Science of the Total Environment, 430*, 75–81. https://doi.org/10.1016/j.scitotenv.2012.04.040.

Zock, J., Zock, J. P., Plana, E., Jarvis, D., Antó, J. M., Kromhout, H., et al. (2007). The use of household cleaning sprays and adult asthma. *American Journal of Respiratory and Critical Care Medicine, 176*(8), 735–741. https://doi.org/10.1164/rccm.200612-1793OC.

Chapter 4
Interactions Among Health Risk Factors and Decision-Making Process in the Design of Built Environments

Abstract The identification of interactions among parameters of health risk factors is a crucial step for the effective assessment and prevention of problems in unhealthy built environments. This chapter introduces the health risk management process in the context of the designs of healthy built environments (Sect. 4.1). In Sects. 4.2–4.3, comprehensive descriptions of all detected interactions among health risks and their parameters that have harmful impacts on user health and wellbeing are defined. Section 4.2 provides a detailed analysis of **single group interactions** between:

- physical-physical,
- chemical-chemical,
- chemical-physical,
- chemical-biological,
- biological-biological,
- biological-physical,
- personal-physical,
- personal-chemical, and
- interactions between other health risk factors and their parameters.

In addition to single group interactions, **multi-group interactions** among health risk factors and their parameters are also analysed in Sect. 4.3. Additionally, synergistic and antagonistic effects are presented, and the main findings are supported by epidemiological studies. The chapter concludes with the tool developed for decision-making processes (Sect. 4.4) supported by the short-term and long-term benefits of holistic design (Sect. 4.5).

M. Dovjak and A. Kukec, *Creating Healthy and Sustainable Buildings*, https://doi.org/10.1007/978-3-030-19412-3_4

4.1   Health Risk and Management Assessment Model in Built Environments

The term "health risk management" describes the process of evaluating alternative regulatory actions and selection among them. It entails the consideration of political, social, economic, and engineering information with risk-related information to develop, analyse, and compare regulatory options and to select the appropriate regulatory response to a potential health hazard (Paustenbach 2002; Yassi et al. 2001).

In the context of built environments, the health risk and management assessment is a dynamic approach. This process of risk and management assessment includes eight main components (Paustenbach 2002; Yassi et al. 2001):

Risk assessment

1. Hazard identification (single group interactions: interactions between two groups of health risk factors and their parameters; multifactorial interactions are interactive influences among parameters of different groups of risk factors),
2. Dose-response assessment (identify relevant toxicity data),
3. Exposure assessment (identification of exposed populations and exposure pathways, direct and indirect methods for assessment values in different sources of identified parameters),
4. Risk characterization (characterize and summarize potential effects of single and/or multifactorial hazards for adverse health).

Risk management

5. Risk evaluation (defined options from different environmental health factors, socio-economic factors, and political aspects),
6. Risk communication (informed decisions),
7. Control and management of exposure (actions to implement the decisions)
8. Risk management strategy (monitoring and evaluate the effectiveness of the action taken).

4.2   Single-Group Interactions

Single group interactions are interactions between **two groups of health risk factors and their parameters**, such as physical-physical, chemical-chemical, chemical-physical, chemical-biological, biological-biological, biological-physical, personal-physical, personal-chemical and interactions between other health risk factors and their parameters.

4.2.1 Physical-Physical Interactions

Detected physical-physical interactions are interactive influences among **parameters of the group of physical risk factors** (Table 4.1).

The first studies on SBS appeared in the 1970s; physical risk factors were primarily examined. The main reasons for this may be related to the introduction of thermal insulated building envelopes, synthetic materials, and the application of mechanical systems. Solutions for lowering energy use were partly defined on the level of thermally improved materials and mechanical systems.

Among physical risk factors, a number of studies examine the correlations between **room air temperature, relative air humidity**, and **ventilation parameters**. Additionally, other parameters of physical risk factors, such as noise, daylight, and electromagnetic fields and ions in relation to SBS were examined in a small number of studies.

Full-scale measurements (Omrani et al. 2017) were performed to investigate the effect of **natural ventilation mode** (i.e., single-sided, cross ventilation) on **thermal comfort and ventilation performance**. Results highlighted a significantly better performance of cross ventilation over single-sided ventilation. Indoor thermal

Table 4.1 Parameters of the group of physical risk factors

Parameters of thermal comfort	• Air temperature, surface temperature, absolute humidity of the air, air velocity, metabolic rate, clothing
Parameters of building ventilation	• Ventilation mode • Qualitative and quantitative parameters of ventilation (e.g., ventilation rate, airflow)
Noise and vibrations	• Sources and noise characteristics, sound level • Parameters related to sound insulation of construction complexes (e.g., weighted apparent sound reduction index, weighted standardized impact sound pressure level) • Room acoustics (e.g., reverberation time) • Vibration frequency, velocity, acceleration
Daylight	• Qualitative and quantitative parameters of daylight for visual and non-visual effects (e.g., illuminance, wavelength, time availability, spatial distribution, etc.)
Electromagnetic fields	• Type and characteristics of sources, distance of the source, radiation protection areas and zones, qualitative and quantitative characteristics of radiation (e.g., electric field strength, magnetic field strength, power density, averaging time, etc.)
Ions	• Sources • Air concentration of positive and negative ions
Ergonomic issues and universal design	• Quantitative and qualitative aspects of task/environment/process/equipment design to fit the worker (dimensions, location, dynamic, static)

conditions were found to be within the comfort zone more than 70% of the time under cross ventilation operation while single-sided ventilation provided adequate thermal conditions only 1% of the time.

In the Report by Commission of the European Communities (ECA 1989), indirect effects of **low relative air humidity** are defined and include **static electricity** and consequent electric discharges and variations of the respirable suspended particulate matter in indoor environments (ECA 1989). Smallwood (2018) determined that static electricity nuisance shocks have become prevalent since floor covering and shoe sole materials have been increasingly made from highly insulating materials, such as polymers. Additionally, the author concluded that atmospheric humidity has a significant role in floor electrical resistance and static charge build-up (Smallwood 2018).

Industrial machines, ventilation machinery, and other **mechanical systems** may produce low-frequency **noise** and **vibrations**. In current design practice, low-frequency noise and vibrations are often neglected, because they are not perceived. Schwartz (2008) highlighted that high-frequency noises—such as telephones, people talking, and computers—can actually mask the effects of low-frequency noise. If mechanical vibrations in the frequency range below 20 Hz (ground-borne vibrations) affect dwelling rooms, the annoying effects are perceived only by a small portion of exposed individuals as a physical effect (Findeis and Peters 2004).

Even if low-frequency noise is not perceived by occupants, it should not be ignored with regards to the health perspective. In the study on office environment by Burt (1996), **low-frequency noise**, produced by **ventilation systems**, was responsible for some of the SBS experienced by the occupants: fatigue, headache, nausea, concentration difficulties, disorientation, motion sickness, digestive disorders, cough, vision problems and dizziness. Burt (1996) concluded that repeated or long-term exposure to such amplified infrasound may trigger an allergic-type response in individuals. Similar findings were found by Hodgson et al. (1987) on vibrations in office environments, showing that an **adjacent pump-room caused vibrations** that resulted in the occurrence of SBS symptoms among a group of secretaries.

4.2.2 Chemical-Chemical Interactions

Detected chemical-chemical interactions are interactive influences **among the parameters of the group of chemical risk factors** (Table 4.2).

Studies on chemical risk factors are mainly focused on the links between SBS symptoms exposure to different emission sources, such as construction products, furniture, and household products. They revealed the possible adverse health effects of construction products on building occupants, during normal use of the building or during emergency situations (i.e. fire). Despite those issues, many construction

Table 4.2 Parameters of the group of chemical risk factors

Construction and household products, furniture, equipment and emitted pollutants	Composition and emission of hazardous chemicals (e.g., formaldehyde, phthalates, volatile organic compounds, etc.)
Odours	Outdoor and indoor sources (i.e., animal farm, landfill, materials, household waste, individual heating, vicinity of industry, busy roads, highways) Composition and concentration Bio-effluents, bioaerosols
Man-made mineral fibre	Man-made vitreous (silicate) fibres: refractory ceramic fibres (RCF), special-purpose glass fibres, glass wool, rock wool, slag wool and continuous glass filaments. Usage according to function (thermal and acoustic insulation), installation, worker prevention Composition and emission of hazardous chemicals
Environmental tobacco smoke	Main-stream or side-stream smoke Number of smokers Used accessories (cigarettes, electronic cigarettes, vaporizers, etc.) Time, period
Biocides	Composition, usage Time, period
Other indoor pollutants	Cleaners, radon (from the ground)

and household products on the market may present potential health concerns. The composition of **construction** and **household products** in relation to the content of **harmful substances** is often questionable; the relevant legislation and inspection are incomplete.

Construction products, household products, furniture, and other equipment may emit harmful substances in the surrounding environment throughout their life cycle (Dovjak and Kristl 2011; Šestan et al. 2013). Wooden construction products and furniture (i.e., plywood, particleboard, fibreboard, oriented strand board (OSB), panel boards, urea-formaldehyde foam, etc.), paints, adhesives, varnishes, floor finishes, disinfectants, cleaning agents, and other household products emit **formaldehyde** (Šestan et al. 2013). In addition to its widespread use in everyday life, formaldehyde (and its health effects) is one of the most examined harmful substances in relation to construction products and indoor air quality issues. Adverse health effects from exposure to formaldehyde in prefabricated houses, especially irritation of the eyes and upper airways, were first reported in the mid-1960s (Salthammer et al. 2010). Current studies are focused on the potential exposure and cancer risk from formaldehyde emissions from installed construction products (Sheehan et al. 2017). A long-term study of formaldehyde emission decay from particle board has been carried out by Zinn et al. (1990). For products manufactured in 1986 and 1987, the overall three-quarter (75% of initial concentration) and half-lives were 38 and 216 days, respectively (Salthammer et al. 2010).

Polyvinyl chloride (PVC) construction products, personal-care products, medical devices, detergents and surfactants, packaging, children's toys, modelling clay, waxes, paints, printing inks and coatings, pharmaceuticals, food products, and textiles contain **phthalates**, which are easily released into the environment because there is no covalent bond between the phthalates and plastics (Dovjak and Kristl 2011). The earliest research about their adverse effects on human health was when Šarić et al. (1976) published the article about malignant tumours of the liver and lungs in an area with the PVC industry. In the 1980s and '90s, the studies were focused primarily on cancer (Heudorf et al. 2007; Jaakkola et al. 1999; Blount et al. 2000). Moreover, studies in the late 1990s concluded that these chemicals are thought to be endocrine disruptors, responsible for low testosterone levels, declining sperm counts and quality, genital malformations, retarded sexual development or even reproductive abnormalities and increased incidences of certain types of cancer (Heudorf et al. 2007; Blount et al. 2000). Currently, the majority of studies (Jaakkola et al. 1999; Bornehag et al. 2004) showed the association between phthalates and asthma, allergies, or related respiratory effects. In the study by Subedi et al. (2017), concentrations of potentially toxic plasticizers (phthalates, non-phthalates) were investigated in 28 dust samples collected from three different indoor environments across the USA. The observed concentrations of these replacement non-phthalate plasticizers were as high as di-(2-ethylhexyl) phthalate, the most frequently detected phthalate plasticizer at the highest concentration worldwide, in most indoor dust samples. The estimated daily intakes of total phthalates (n = 7) by children and toddlers through indoor dust in childcare facilities were 1.6 times higher than the non-phthalate plasticizers (n = 3), whereas the estimated daily intake of total non-phthalates for all age groups at homes were 1.9 times higher than the phthalate plasticizers. Occupational intake of phthalate and non-phthalate plasticizers through the indoor dust at hair salons was more elevated than at homes in the USA.

In addition to plasticizers, **flame retardants** are used in a variety of **construction products** and **furniture**. Takeuchi et al. (2014) measured 59 compounds, including plasticizers (phthalates, adipates, and others) and flame retardants (organo-phosphates and brominated compounds), from indoor air samples from six houses in Sapporo, Japan. Among the 59 compounds measured in this study, 34 were detected from the indoor air of the six houses. These results suggested that compounds with higher volatility exist preferentially in the gas phase, whereas compounds with lower volatility exist preferentially in the particulate phase in indoor air.

Volatile organic compounds (VOCs) are emitted as gases from certain solids or liquids. VOCs include a variety of chemicals, some of which may have short- and long-term adverse health effects. Concentrations of many VOCs are consistently higher indoors (up to ten times higher) than outdoors (EPA 2017). Sources of VOCs in indoor environments include construction products, furniture, household products (waxes, detergent, insecticides), products of personal hygiene (cosmetics), do-it-yourself goods (resins), office materials (photocopier ink) or ETS (ECA 1989). A cross-sectional epidemiological study by Azuma et al. (2017) examined the correlation between indoor air quality and building-related symptoms of office workers (N = 107 office workers during winter, 207 office workers during summer) in 17 air-conditioned office buildings in Tokyo, Osaka, and Fukuoka. The study found that several irritating VOCs (e.g., formaldehyde, acetaldehyde, ethylbenzene, toluene, and xylenes) that were positively correlated with the indoor air concentration among their VOCs were associated with upper respiratory symptoms, although their indoor air concentrations were lower than those specified by the indoor air quality guidelines.

Inefficient ventilation systems, incomplete combustion processes, unvented heating, gas cooking, tobacco smoking may result in higher concentrations of other indoor air quality (IAQ) pollutants such as CO_2, CO, NO_X, SO_X (ECA 1989). IAQ pollutants may present a significant source of **odours** (ECA 1989, Nakaoka et al. 2014), natural (e.g., users, animals, plants, etc.) or artificial origin (e.g., materials, systems, etc.). Odours are organic or inorganic compounds and can be both pleasant and unpleasant. Some odours can be health hazards, and some are not (CDC 2017).

Users emit **bio-effluents** (volatile and non-volatile organic compound) and **bioaerosols** (particles) (Bivolarova et al. 2017). The most commonly known bio-effluent produced by human metabolism is CO_2. Bioaerosols may consist of bacteria, fungi (and spores and cell fragments of fungi), viruses, microbial toxins, pollen, plant fibres, etc. (Douwes et al. 2003). Qualitative and quantitative characterization of bio-effluents and bioaerosols should be considered in the design of ventilation systems.

4.2.3 Chemical-Physical Interactions

Detected chemical-physical interactions are interactive influences among **parameters of the group of chemical risk factors and parameters of the group of physical risk factors** (parameters of thermal comfort, parameters related to building ventilation systems, noise, vibrations, daylight, EM fields, ions, ergonomic issues, universal design).

The emission rates of harmful substances from the construction products, household products, furniture, and other indoor sources are influenced by environmental conditions, such as air temperature, surface temperatures, relative humidity of indoor air, air change rate and surface air velocity (ECA 1989; Haghighat et al. 1998; Sakai et al. 2004; Järnström et al. 2006; Blondel and Plaisance 2011; Clausen et al. 2012; Kim et al. 2012; Xu et al. 2009; Nimmermark and Gustafsson 2005). The impact of environmental parameters on the emission behaviours of various compounds was studied in laboratory conditions inside a test chamber or in real built environments. Huang et al. (2015) proved that **relative humidity** is one of the main environmental factors affecting the emission behaviours of **formaldehyde** from construction products. The results of their experimental study showed that formaldehyde emissions increased by 10 times as relative humidity increased from 20 to 85%. Xu and Zhang (2011) found the opposite, concluding that there is no distinguishable difference in the effective diffusion coefficient of formaldehyde when the relative humidity is between 25 and 50%.

Sakai et al. (2004) performed a comparative study in urban dwellings in Japan and Sweden and proved that indoor concentrations of **formaldehyde** were increased at higher **air temperature** and **relative humidity**. The same findings were reported in the study by Järnström et al. (2006) for new residential buildings in Finland and in the study by Blondel and Plaisance (2011) for students' rooms in France. Järnström et al. (2006) measured higher concentrations of formaldehyde in summer, at higher air temperatures and relative humidity. Vice versa, lower concentrations were measured in winter, at lower air temperatures and drier air. Blondel and Plaisance (2011) concluded that the rise of formaldehyde emissions from indoor materials correlated with air temperature. Similar findings were confirmed in an experimental study in a test chamber by Zhang et al. (2007), where the increase of air temperature resulted in higher emission rates of formaldehyde from analysed materials.

In addition to air temperature and relative humidity, **air velocity** also has an important effect on the emissions of indoor materials. In a study by Zhu et al. (2013), the effect of ventilation on the **VOCs concentration** was analysed by using the developed integrated model for VOCs emission/sorption from/on building materials. The results showed that concentration in the air varies with the same tendency as the air exchange rate.

Pollutant emissions are also related to the type of **HVAC system**. Chen et al. (2016) studied formaldehyde emissions from porous building material under non-isothermal conditions. Experiments demonstrating the emission of formaldehyde during floor heating and air circulation systems were carried out in a controlled environmental chamber. The results showed that the equilibrium concentration in an airtight chamber with a floor heating system is higher than that in an air circulation heating system.

In addition to formaldehyde emissions, **air temperature** and **relative humidity** have a significant effect on the emissions of other indoor air pollutants, such as **phthalates, VOCs and odours**. Clausen et al. (2012) analysed the influences of air temperature and relative humidity on the emission of di-(2-ethylhexyl) phthalate (DEHP) from PVC flooring. The study concluded that **DEHP concentrations** increased substantially with increasing **air temperature** and were independent of the relative humidity. Similarly, the study by Nimmermark and Gustafsson (2005) showed that **odour emission** increased significantly with **air temperature** at constant ventilation rates. A comprehensive literature review by Haghighat et al. (1998) noted that emission rates of total volatile organic compounds (**TVOCs**) increased with **air temperature** for both paint and varnish. However, the individual compounds did not necessarily follow the same trend established by the TVOC; they showed greater emission rates at lower air temperatures. The effects of relative humidity on the emissions of TVOC differed between paint and varnish. Individual compounds showed higher emission rates for lower levels of humidity and vice versa. The VOC emission characteristics of these materials are essential for understanding indoor air pollution dynamics (Jiang et al. 2017). Jiang et al. (2017) investigated the emission characteristics of VOCs from particleboard in sealed or ventilated environmental chambers at different temperatures (23, 35, or 50 °C), with a focus on the emission of odorous compounds. The emissions of **HCHO** and **total VOCs** (TVOC) from the particleboard increased significantly with **temperature**, and the emitted VOC mixtures had complex chemical compositions. At room temperature (23 °C), n-hexane was the most abundant compound, except HCHO; but at higher temperatures, concentrations of **hexanal** and **pentanal** significantly increased. Moreover, due to their low **odour** thresholds, aldehydes, particularly hexanal and pentanal, were identified as the major odorous compounds emitted from the particleboard.

In addition to air temperature and relative humidity, **VOC emissions** are influenced by **surface temperatures**. Kim et al. (2012) measured VOC emissions from building materials in residential buildings in Korea with radiant floor heating systems. The results showed that the **VOC emissions** from flooring materials increased as the **floor temperature** rises. In particular, increased temperatures may accelerate chemical reactions within the material, leading to additional VOC emissions (Kim et al. 2012). Emitted pollutants can be adsorbed onto indoor surfaces (carpet, wood, skin) and re-emit in indoor air (Xu et al. 2009) or they may react with each other and form secondary pollutants.

High **relative humidity** in combination with **room temperatures** often results in dampness and **odours**. Dampness-related problems (i.e., mould spots, damp stains, water damage and condensation) are risk factors for the perceptions of odours and sensations of humid air and dry air, as proven by Wang et al. (2013), in domestic environments in Chongqing, China and Zhang et al. (2012) in workplace buildings in Uppsala, Sweden.

The **type of building ventilation system** (i.e., natural-ventilation vs. mechanical systems) was related to **IAQ and SBS** as it was presented in the comparative study by Costa and Brickus (2000) in Niteroi, Rio de Janeiro, Brazil. Occupants in naturally ventilated offices have fewer SBS symptoms than occupants of air-conditioned offices (Costa and Brickus 2000, Seppänen and Fisk 2002). The importance of effective household ventilation via window opening frequency in the prevention of the negative effects of home dampness exposure on common cold was highlighted in the study by Sun et al. (2017). A cross-sectional survey on home environment and childhood health collected 13,335 parent-reported questionnaires of 4–6-year-old children in Shanghai, China. The results revealed that dampness-related exposures and household ventilation habits (p-value for interaction <0.001) had a strong interaction effect on the incidence and duration of the common cold.

In a field experiment by Shan et al. (2016), two identical tutorial rooms were studied to compare **human subjects' thermal comfort, SBS**, and **short-term performance** under **mixing ventilation** and **passive displacement ventilation**.

Higher CO_2 concentration was the main factor causing SBS related to the head, while both higher CO_2 concentration and lower relative humidity contributed to SBS related to the eyes. As a consequence, SBS resulted from high CO_2 concentration and low relative humidity could lead to decrease in short-term performance. Mixing ventilation leads to higher overall draft sensation while displacement ventilation results in the sensation of cold feet.

Inadequately functioning, obsolete, and poorly maintained HVAC systems, decreased number of air changes, and decreased volumes of clean air may lead to increased concentrations of indoor air pollutants and may result in the occurrence of SBS symptoms (ECA 1989; Redlich et al. 1997; Assimakopoulos and Helmis 2004; Seppänen et al. 1999). Moreover, ventilation rates strongly influence the emission rates from indoor sources, such as DEHP emission rates from PVC flooring. Similar findings were reported in a study by Hodgson (2000) in houses in Florida, where **VOCs emission rates** at the low and high **ventilation rates** decreased with decreasing compound volatility. Additionally, the ventilation system itself can be a source of air pollutants. Unsealed fibreglass and other insulation material lining the ventilation ducts can release particulate material into the air. Such material can also become wet, creating an ideal and often concealed site for the growth of microorganisms (Redlich et al. 1997). Azuma et al. (2017) studied the correlation between indoor pollutants and building-related symptoms on office workers (N = 107 workers during winter, 207 workers during summer) in 17 buildings with air-conditioning systems in Tokyo, Osaka, and Fukuoka. Results revealed that upper respiratory symptoms showed a significant correlation with increased indoor temperatures and increased indoor concentrations of suspended particles released from the ambient air pollution via air-conditioning systems during winter.

Construction products can affect the transport and removal of indoor **VOCs by sorption and desorption**. Zhu et al. (2013) developed an integrated model capable of predicting the emission/sorption of VOCs from/on building materials under variable air exchange rates. Construction products can act as sinks or sources of VOCs emission.

4.2.4 Chemical-Biological Interactions

Chemical-biological interactions are interactive influences **among parameters of the group of chemical risk factors** and **parameters of the group of biological risk factors** (i.e., moulds, bacteria, MVOCs, house dust).

Household dust serves as a good proxy for assessing indoor air pollution (Gustafsson et al. 2018). A characterization of residential house-dust by Gustafsson et al. (2018) showed that the respirable fraction of dust contains aluminium and zinc as dominating metals, silicon dioxide and calcium carbonate as the major mineral components, and bacterial, fungi and skin fragments in an organic matrix.

House dust often contains substances that are emitted from construction products, i.e., **phthalate esters** and other plasticisers emitted from PVC products (Kishi et al. 2012; Bamai et al. 2014), brominated flame retardants (Kajiwara and Takigami 2016), etc. Bamai et al. (2016) estimated **phthalate intake** from urinary metabolite among Japanese children and **house dust levels** in living environment. The results suggested that, among Japanese children, house dust from low surfaces, such as living room floors, might play a meaningful role in the indoor environmental exposure pathway for BBzP and DEHP. Phthalate intake via dust ingestion seems more strongly related to health than total intake.

Polybrominated diphenyl ethers (PBDEs) and **hexabromocyclododecanes (HBCDs)** are widely used as synthetic additives to reduce the flammability of plastics, textile coatings, and electronic appliances (Kajiwara and Takigami 2016). Although the use of PBDEs and HBCDs has been phased out as per international regulations, they still contribute greatly to the overall emissions. Kajiwara and Takigami (2016) examined the concentrations, profiles, and mass distributions of polybrominated diphenyl ethers (PBDEs), hexabromocyclododecanes (HBCDs), and polybrominated dibenzo-p-dioxins/furans (PBDD/Fs) based on the particle sizes of **house dust samples** from five homes in Japan. PBDEs, HBCDs, and PBDFs were detected in all the samples analysed.

A direct or indirect relation between damp or mould in the home and respiratory health were examined by Peat et al. (1998). **Home dampness** is thought to have health consequences because it has the potential to increase the proliferation of **house-dust mites** and **moulds**, both of which are allergens.

4.2.5 Biological-Biological Interactions

In the 1980s, in addition to physical risk factors, a number of studies examined biological risk factors, specifically the association between the presence of many biological agents in the indoor environment and dampness-related problems (mould spots, damp stains, water damage, and condensation) as well as inadequate ventilation. Studies on the exposure to other biological risk factors and SBS occurrence are scarce at present, mainly due to the fact that SBS but also BRI presents a common result of exposure to biological agents (i.e., aspergillosis).

Biological-biological interactions are interactive influences **among parameters of the group of biological risk factors** (Table 4.3).

The major sources of micro-organisms in indoor environment areas are humans, pets, room plants, waste, house dust, textiles, carpets, furniture fillers, and air filters

Table 4.3 Parameters of the group of biological risk factors

Bacteria	*Micrococcus* sp., *Staphylococcus* sp., *Streptococcus* sp., *Bacillus* sp., *Neisseria* sp., *Actinomyces* sp. (Sekulska et al. 2007)
Moulds	*Cladosporium* sp., *Penicillium* sp., *Aspergillus* sp., *Mucor* sp. (Yassin and Almouqatea 2010; Sekulska et al. 2007)
Viruses	Many viruses that infect humans (respiratory tract, common cold, e.g., Adenoviruses, influenza e.g., influenza viruses)

for HVAC systems that are not properly maintained or not replaced in time (Yassin and Almouqatea 2010).

The association between **MVOCs, dampness, and mould** was reported in the study by Assimakopoulos and Helmis (2004) on a public building in the centre of Athens and in the study by Sahlberg et al. (2013) in 159 homes in Reykjavik, Uppsala and Tartu. Opposite findings were found in a study by Wieslander et al. (2007) on health effects in office workers (N = 18) in a medical casebook archive with dampness caused by flooding. The measurements of moulds and microbial volatile organic compounds could not identify any obvious exposure contrast between the damp building and the dry control building. The flooded building had slightly higher levels of MVOC. However, subjects previously exposed to building dampness had an increase of symptoms.

Examination of MVOCs in indoor air has also become an important method for the detection of the type and intensity of masked contamination by moulds (Fiedler et al. 2001; Choi et al. 2017).

4.2.6 Biological-Physical Interactions

Detected biological-physical interactions are interactive influences **among parameters of the group of biological risk factors** and **parameters of the group of physical risk factors.**

High relative air humidity in combination with air temperature may lead to the occurrence of condensation on surfaces, material damage, dampness, and toxic mould growth (ECA, 1989).

Moisture and temperature are the two key environmental parameters that determine the possibility of **mould growth on construction complexes** (Sautour et al. 2002). At relative humidity at or above 75–80% (0.75–0.8 water activity, water available in the material for microbial growth,), there is a possible risk of mould growth on construction products (Grant et al. 1989; Johansson et al. 2013). Relative humidity is affected by temperature, as temperature is reduced below 5 or increased above 35 °C (Zak and Wildman 2004), cellular processes are slowed down. In addition to air temperature and relative humidity, the type of material and its specific critical moisture level are important influential factors. If this is exceeded, there is a risk that mould fungi will develop on the material.

In indoor active spaces, the temperature and relative humidity often fluctuate due to seasonal variations, user activities, etc. The effect of **cyclic moisture and temperature** on mould growth on wood compared to steady-state conditions was studied by Johansson et al. (2013). The authors proved that the duration of favourable conditions of relative humidity was decisive for mould growth and fluctuating temperature lead to slower mould growth. Additionally, the impact of moisture content in construction products on mould growth is presented in more detail in Sect. 4.4.

In a study by Lappalainen et al. (2015), **VOC emissions from hidden mould** growth were investigated using an IAQ simulator test. **MVOCs** can be released from a moisture-damaged wall structure into an indoor environment, and the impact of the **relative humidity of the material** is remarkable. The concentration of **MVOC** is also related to **absolute humidity** and **ventilation efficiency**. A case-control investigation (198 cases and 202 controls) showed that homes with a high concentration of the MVOC were not only associated with a high absolute humidity but were also poorly ventilated. Specifically, joint exposure to high MVOCs and high absolute humidity was associated with 2.6-times greater odds of the doctor-diagnosed childhood asthma (95% CI, 0.7–8.91; P = 0.137).

Additionally, **mites** as important biological agents are related to a **room's relative humidity**. They can be destroyed by keeping absolute humidity below 7 g/kg of air (about 45%) during the winter time (ECA 1989). If relative humidity is too low, which usually happens during the heating season, humidifiers are introduced. Humidifiers provide an optimal place for microbes to flourish. In addition to humidifiers, dehumidifiers, cooling devices, indoor A/C units are problematic for the growth of microorganisms (ECA 1989).

Salimifard et al. (2017) investigated the impacts of **humidity** and **air swirl** on the resuspension of **biological particles** (i.e., quartz, dust mite, cat fur, dog fur, and bacterial spore-*Bacillus thuringiensis* as an anthrax simulant) from floor and duct surfaces. The results showed that the **particle property** of being hydrophilic or hydrophobic plays an important role in the particle resuspension rate. The resuspension rates of hydrophilic **dust mite** particles increase up to two orders of magnitude as **relative humidity** decreased from 80 to 10% at 25 °C. However, the resuspension rates of cat fur and dog fur particles that are hydrophobic are within the measurement error range (±15%) over 10–80% relative humidity. With regard to the resuspension of bacterial spores (*Bacillus thuringiensis*) from a duct surface, the resuspension rates are substantially affected by air swirl velocity and particle size (Salimifard et al. 2017).

Human-made water systems (e.g., hot water systems, ventilation systems, cooling towers, humidifiers, whirlpool spas) are common sources of outbreaks of *Legionella* **infection** (NIPH 2012). Transmission can also occur in public and residential buildings. Incidence of the disease is higher in the summertime, possibly because of increased use of cooling towers for air conditioning systems and differences in water chemistry when **outdoor temperatures** are higher (Prussin et al. 2017).

Major **indoor environmental factors**, such as relative humidity, characteristics of air ventilation systems, seasonal variation, temperature, and chemical composition of the air influencing **bioaerosol concentration** (Law et al. 2001; Park et al. 2001). Studies proved (Law et al. 2001; Park et al. 2001) that concentrations of **endotoxin and airborne fungi** were positively related to **indoor relative humidity** (higher concentration associated with higher relative humidity). Relative humidity also affects the infectivity of airborne viruses (Verreault et al. 2008).

4.2.7 Personal-Physical Interactions

In the 1990s, researchers realized that SBS was influenced also by psychosocial, personal, and other risk factors. Nevertheless, psychosocial, personal and other risk factors remain neglected research areas.

> Detected physical-personal interactions are interactive influences **among parameters of the group of physical risk factors** and **parameters of the group personal risk factors** (gender, health status, individual differences).

A literature survey on how different factors influence human comfort in indoor environments (Frontczak and Wargocki 2011) showed that thermal comfort was influenced by the level of education, the relationship with superiors and colleagues and time pressure, but not by gender, age, body build, fitness, health, self-estimated environmental sensitivity, menstruation cycle, pattern of smoking and coffee drinking, job stress or hours worked per week. Additionally, the impact of individuality on thermal sensation was presented in greater detail in Chaps. 1 and 2.

Social status is a significant health determinant related to built environments. Several studies (Metin Özcan et al. 2013; Yun and Steemers 2011; Santamouris et al. 2007) evaluated the association between social status and indoor environmental quality issues. The considered socio-economic indicator in these studies was fuel poverty.

BOX 4.1 Fuel poverty

A person is to be regarded as living "in fuel poverty" if he is a member of a household living on a lower income in a home that cannot be kept warm at a reasonable cost (WHECA 2000). A frequently used definition is that when a household needs to spend more than 10% of its income to keep its dwelling adequately warm and for other energy services, it is fuel poor (Boardmann 1991).

Fuel poverty is measured by:

- inability to keep homes adequately warm,
- arrears on utility bills,
- people living in a dwelling with a leaking roof, damp walls, floors or foundation (Kontonasiou et al. 2015).

Between 50 and 125 million people in the EU are estimated to suffer from fuel poverty (WHO 2012). The number will inevitably rise in the future as global energy prices increase (EPEE 2017). The data from the Assessment report on environmental health inequalities in Europe (WHO 2012) provide strong evidence that the non-sanitary housing inequalities—overcrowding, dampness and thermal comfort related to cool and warm homes—exist in almost every country. Similar results were found in a Pan-European study (Velux 2016; Velux Group 2017), Europeans who live in energy poverty are almost three times as likely to live in damp, unhealthy buildings.

Low-income populations, and especially low-income single-parent households and the elderly are the most affected across all indicators.

Fuel poverty is strongly related to ability to keep a home comfortably warm in winter and comfortably cool in summer (WHO 2012; BPIE 2014). Forty-five percent of the studied European population reduce their temperatures to lower their energy bills (Velux 2016). In addition to winter, summer indoor air temperatures may be a problem. The proportion of the general population unable to keep their dwellings comfortably cool in summer is even higher than the proportion unable to keep the home warm in winter (WHO 2012).

The increasing trend of fuel poverty is related to indoor environmental quality issues. In 2012, 12.9% of the EU-28 population declared that their dwelling was not comfortably warm during winter, and almost 20.0% of Europeans perceived their dwellings to be not sufficiently insulated against excessive heat during summer (Eurostat 2017).

The environmental health inequalities in relation to built environment issues represent critical research areas on the global and national scales. Findings on the association between socio-economic indicators and indoor environmental quality are beneficial especially in defining national laws on housing and social policies as well as defining priority actions to ensure their effective implementation throughout the country.

For example, in 2015, households in Slovenia spent on average 6.7% of their disposable income on electricity, gas and other fuels, which is 0.7 of a percentage point less than in 2012 (latest available data) and the same as in 2000. Having reviewed the distribution of households by income quintiles, we found that expenditure for electricity, gas and other fuels in 2015 in the first quintile (representing 20% of households with the lowest income) represented on average 17.7%. Fuel poverty indicators among people at risk of poverty in Slovenia are: 37.5% arrears on utility bills (10% EU average), 17.3% inability to keep home adequately warm (10.8% EU average) and 46.1% dwellings with leakages & damp walls

(15.1% EU average) (Kontonasiou et al. 2015). Socio-economic status is related to indoor environmental quality issues. The results of the online pilot survey in Slovenia on 714 respondents (Recek 2017; Recek et al. 2019) showed that households with a better socio-economic status spend more household income for a better living comfort and consequently stay in facilities with better indoor environmental quality. Such environmental quality is also detected in buildings with higher energy efficiency. Based on the results of the online survey, the socio-economic status of a household does not influence the energy efficiency of a building. The main reason for the investment in increased energy efficiency of buildings is lower energy consumption for heating, to which respondents give priority over indoor environmental quality (Recek 2017; Recek et al. 2019).

4.2.8 Personal-Chemical Interactions

The most important findings of the literature review show that many studies have examined the correlation between SBS symptoms and physical risk factors as well as the correlation between SBS symptoms and chemical risk factors, while the evidence on the correlation between SBS symptoms and biological, psychological, personal and other risk factors is for the moment scarce.

> Detected personal-chemical interactions are interactive influences **among parameters of the group of personal risk factors** and **parameters of the group of chemical risk factors.**

Many studies have focused on the adverse health effects of indoor air pollutants among highly sensitive groups of individuals, such as children, the elderly, and occupational groups (Heudorf et al. 2007; Jaakkola et al. 1999).

Numerous epidemiological studies have shown associations between air pollution and reduced lung function and increased prevalence of respiratory diseases among children and young adults (Sierra-Vargas and Teran 2012). Current epidemiological studies that explore the impact of indoor air quality on respiratory diseases are mostly limited to estimations of prevalence or incidence observed in a particular age group (Eder et al. 2006). Due to their physiological characteristics, children are vulnerable in relation to environmental impact, as they inhale more air than adults do and, therefore, their exposure is greater. Toxic substances may disrupt or interfere with the rapid development of various body functions, which can lead to irreversible diseases and organ damage. Indoor pollutants can cause or aggravate various medical conditions such as allergies, asthma, and other respiratory diseases. Thus, a healthy school environment is crucial in protecting the health of children since they spend up to eight hours per day and nine months per year in the school premises (WHO 2004). The number of studies exploring the association between respiratory diseases and indoor air quality is increasing although the number of studies in educational institutions remains relatively low, as most epidemiological research focuses on indoor air at home. One indicator of respiratory disease is reduced lung function, which can be measured with spirometry. In this procedure, the volume and rate of exhaled air is measured, from which the state of illness in the respiratory tract may be inferred (Kaminsky 2012). Asthma is the most common childhood disease in developed countries with a statistically significant morbidity and increasing prevalence (Eder et al. 2006). Typical symptoms are bronchial hyper-responsiveness, chronic inflammation of the airways, and recurrent wheezing (Weichenthal et al. 2007). The identification of air pollutants that are causally associated with the development of asthma is extremely difficult due to the complex combination of pollutants and etiological heterogeneity of asthma (Delfino 2002).

The positive correlation between oxidative stress, indoor air pollution (VOC, CO_2), and SBS complaints was proved in the study by Lu et al. (2007) among 389 office workers in 87 government offices of eight high-rise buildings in Taipei, Taiwan.

4.2.9   Interactions Between Other Health Risk Factors and Their Parameters

The strong relationship between **ownership** and **building age** was proved by Engvall et al. (2000) in Stockholm, 609 multi-family buildings with 14,235 dwellings. Subjects owning their own building reported less SBS, but 5% of all buildings built before 1961, 13% of those built in 1976-1984, and 15% of those built in 1985–1990 would have significantly more SBS than expected. Mizoue et al. (2001) examined these relations using data from a 1998 cross-sectional survey of 1,281 municipal employees who worked in a variety of buildings in a Japanese city. **Working overtime** for 30 or more hours per month was also associated with SBS symptoms. **Personal lifestyles** are an additional factor.

The association between **personal and psychosocial factors** was confirmed in the study by Ooi and Goh (1997). The authors found an incremental trend in prevalence of SBS among office workers who reported high levels of **physical and mental stress** and **decreasing climate of co-operation**. Similar findings were reported in the study by Burge (2004), where SBS symptoms were generally more common and more problematic in the **stressed**, the **unloved**, and in **individuals who feel powerless to change their situation** (Burge 2004). Another important issue is related to possibility of **individual regulation** and **control of indoor environmental parameters**. Poor individual control of temperature and lighting are associated with increased symptoms (Jaakkola et al. 1989). The study by Burge (2004) proved a strong association between lack of control of the office environment and symptoms. Two quantitative studies (Temeljotov Salaj et al. 2015; Baričič et al. 2014) on 1,036 office workers in Slovenia and 394 office workers in Lebanon showed that real-estate factors of the workspace—in terms of the assessment of

office building and the position of the employee, as well as the workspace design—
have an impact on the satisfaction of employees and, consequently, their assessment
of health.

4.3 Multi-group Interactions

Detected multifactorial interactions are interactive influences among **parameters of different groups of risk factors.** Many studies have analysed
the association between various risk factors for SBS.

The effect of **physical, chemical** and **personal** health risk factors and their
parameters were analysed by Burge (2004). Burge (2004) found out that there was
an association between increasing **air temperature, overcrowding, and inadequate ventilation** and the occurrence of SBS. Household **formaldehyde** exposure
and its associations with **dwelling characteristics, lifestyle behaviours,** and
childhood health outcomes in Shanghai, China was studied by Huang et al.
(2017). Examining 409 children's bedrooms, the authors determined that bedrooms
with mechanical ventilation had lower formaldehyde concentrations than those with
natural ventilation. Results indicated that household formaldehyde exposure may
increase the risk of the common cold in childhood. Household formaldehyde had
few significant associations with the studied illnesses. Families with sick children
perhaps pay more attention to improving indoor air quality.

The effect of **physical, chemical** and **microbiological** characteristics of 19
governmental office buildings in the Netherlands and SBS were analysed by
Teeuw et al. (1994). Moreover, Skov et al. (1990) performed a multivariate logistic
regression analyses on 2,369 office workers in 14 buildings in Copenhagen,
Denmark, in which the influence of various factors, such as the **concentration of
macromolecular organic floor dust, the floor covering, the number of workplaces in the office, the age of the building, the type of ventilation, shelf factor
and fleece factor** on SBS symptoms was investigated.

The effect of **physical, chemical, biological and personal factors** was also
evaluated in **residential buildings.** Lu et al. (2016) studied associations between
**outdoor air pollution, meteorological parameters, and selected indoor expo-
sure** and **building characteristics** at home and weekly SBS symptoms in a standardized questionnaire study among 3,485 randomly selected adults in China.
Indoor factors played a major role in SBS symptoms. Mould/dampness on the floor/
ceiling was associated with fatigue OR = 1.60 (1.11–2.30) and headache OR = 1.80
(1.07–3.04). Mouldy odour was associated with fatigue OR = 1.59 (1.07–2.37) and
dermal symptoms OR = 1.91 (1.21–3.02). Windowpane condensation in winter
was associated with fatigue OR = 1.73 (1.30–2.31) and throat symptoms
OR = 1.53 (1.01–2.31). Damp bed clothing was related with throat symptom

OR = 1.62 (1.09–2.40). Home redecoration was associated with fatigue OR = 1.49 (1.07–2.06). Frequent window opening was associated with less nose symptoms OR = 0.54 (0.36–0.82), and mechanical ventilation in the bathroom reduced dermal symptoms OR = 0.66 (0.44–0.99). Females were more susceptible to redecoration and windowpane condensation than men were. No associations with SBS were observed for outdoor air pollutants or meteorological parameters in the final models combining indoor and outdoor factors, although SO_2, temperature, and relative humidity were associated with some SBS symptoms (fatigue, eyes and nose symptoms) in the separate outdoor models. In conclusion, indoor mould/dampness, air pollution from redecoration, and poorer ventilation conditions in dwellings can be risk factors for SBS symptoms in an adult Chinese population, especially among females (Lu et al. 2016).

The effect of **personal, physical,** and **biological factors** was also statistically evaluated on a **larger scale.** The EU SILC survey (Ecofys 2017) on 100,000 individual households and more than 250,000 adults (16 years and older) proved statistically very significant correlations among **socio-economic indicators, state of building,** and **health issues.** Around 33% of adults (16.2 million) report dampness when being unable to keep their dwelling warm, but only 12% when being able to do so. The probability that adults report dampness is 2.8 times higher when they are unable to keep their dwelling warm. In multi-family buildings, this probability is around 2.5 times higher, and in single-family buildings, this probability is approximately three times higher in comparison to when there are no difficulties. A share of 13% of adults (6.4 million) report lack of daylight when being unable to keep their dwelling warm, but only 6% when being able to do so; 20% of adults (10 million) report poor health when being unable to keep their dwelling warm, but only 9% when being able to do so.

Several studies make the same conclusions that it is difficult to pinpoint the causative factor for SBS due to **multifactorial effects**. In a study of an air-conditioned building in Niteroi, Rio de Janeiro, Brazil, Costa and Brickus (2000) concluded that **poor individual control of temperature** and **lighting** are associated with increased symptoms. A univariate analysis, performed by Abdel-Hamid et al. (2013) at the Faculty of Medicine, Ain Shams University, Cairo, Egypt showed that **poor lighting, poor ventilation, lack of sunlight, absence of air currents, high noise, temperature, humidity, environmental tobacco smoke, use of photocopiers,** and **inadequate office cleaning** were statistically associated with SBS symptoms. Building characteristics, such as **year of construction** and **the effect of indoor emissions** lead to SBS. New houses and new furniture result in higher emissions (Takigawa et al. 2012).

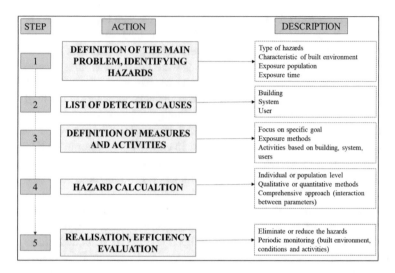

Fig. 4.1 General decision-making process in built environment

4.4 Decision-Making Tool in the Design of Built Environments

The identification of risk factors and their parameters is a crucial step for effective prevention and control of health outcomes in the built environments. Additionally, it is important to detect all interactive influences among factors and their parameters. Detected interactive influences among parameters are problematic fields that have to be eliminated or minimized.

BOX 4.2 Problematic field

A problematic field represents a main focus point in the decision-making process. Specifically, it includes:

– single or multi-group interactions between parameters in built environment,
– exposure time,
– exposure population, especially vulnerable population groups.

For every problematic field, causes and consequences are defined, which serve as a basis for the development of effective measures, accompanied by step-by-step activities to be used in the decision-making process in the design of built environments (Fig. 4.1).

BOX 4.3 Decision-making in the design of built environments

Decision making is the process of identifying the likely consequences of decisions, establishing the importance of single and multi-group interactions between health risk factors, to select the best course of action, to protect user's health in built environment. It should be included in all steps of building design.

Following the evidence-based design approach, the total of 527 sources of literature (Table 4.4) were analysed and presented in previous chapters. As a synthesis, a tool for decision-making process is developed.

BOX 4.4 Evidence-based design approach

The Center for Health Design (CHD) defines evidence-based design approach as "the deliberate attempt to base building decisions on the best available research evidence with the goal of improving outcomes and of continuing to monitor the success or failure for subsequent decision-making." An evidence-based model can be used for all design decisions (Malkin 2008).

The tool is shaped in the form of a matrix, a rectangular array of numbers, symbols, or expressions, arranged in rows and columns. According to our primary goal, to design a healthy built environment with mastered health risk factors and their parameters, altogether six groups of health risk factors and 23 parameters are arranged in rows and columns (Fig. 4.2). Interactive influences among parameters are marked separately in at the crossing points between rows and columns, positioned in the middle of the matrix. For example, cell 9-1 presents the detected interactive influence between physical and chemical health hazard factors, specifically air temperature and formaldehyde emissions from materials (described more in detail in Sect. 4.2).

A detected interactive influence represents a potential problem field that has to be eliminated or minimized. For every marked cell, step-by-step activities for effective prevention and control of health risk factors and their parameters have to be defined. Planned activities should be considered for all possible influences of other factors and parameters (i.e., positive or negative). In such a way, the matrix

Table 4.4 Analysis of relevant sources of literature

Literature type	Number of reviewed references
Scientific study	313
Monograph	57
Scientific report, statistics	103
Regulation, directive, standard, guideline	54
Total	527

Column headers (1–23): 1 T_{ai}, T_{surf}; 2 RH_{ai}; 3 Ventilation parameters; 4 Noise, vibrations; 5 Daylight; 6 EM fields, ions; 7 Ergonomic, universal design; 8 Products, furniture, equipment; 9 HCHO; 10 VOCs; 11 Phthalates; 12 Odours; 13 ETS; 14 MMMF; 15 Biocides; 16 Other pollutants; 17 Moulds; 18 Bacteria; 19 MVOC; 20 House dust; 21 Gender, age, working position; 22 Social status; 23 Other

		Physical								Chemical								Biological				Psychological, personal, other		
		1	2	3	4	5	6	7	8	9	10	11	12	13	14	15	16	17	18	19	20	21	22	23
Physical	1 T_{ai}, T_{surf}	1-1	1-2	1-3		1-5		1-7	1-8	1-9	1-10	1-11	1-12	1-13	1-14	1-15	1-16	1-17	1-18					
	2 RH_{ai}	2-1	2-2	2-3		2-5	2-6	2-7	2-8	2-9	2-10	2-11	2-12			2-15	2-16	2-17	2-18	2-19	2-20			
	3 Ventilation parameters	3-1	3-2	3-3	3-4	3-5	3-6	3-7	3-8	3-9	3-10	3-11	3-12	3-13	3-14	3-15	3-16	3-17	3-18	3-19	3-20	3-21		
	4 Noise, vibrations			4-3	4-4				4-8															
	5 Daylight	5-1					5-6	5-7	5-8															
	6 EM fields, ions		6-2	6-3					6-8															
	7 Ergonomic, universal design	7-1	7-2	7-3	7-4	7-5	7-6	7-7																
	8 Products, furniture, equipment	8-1	8-2	8-3	8-4	8-5	8-6	8-7	8-8	8-9	8-10	8-11	8-12	8-13	8-14	8-15	8-16	8-17	8-18	8-19	8-20			
Chemical	9 HCHO	9-1	9-2	9-3					9-8	9-9			9-12	9-13										
	10 VOCs	10-1	10-2	10-3					10-8		10-10		10-12	10-13										
	11 Phthalates	11-1	11-2	11-3					11-8			11-11									11-20			
	12 Odours	12-1	12-2	12-3					12-8	12-9	12-10		12-12	12-13			12-16	12-17	12-18	12-19				
	13 ETS			13-3					13-8	13-9	13-10		13-12	13-13			13-16					13-21	13-22	
	14 MMMF			14-3					14-8						14-14									
	15 Biocides		15-2	15-3					15-8							15-15		15-17	15-18					
	16 Other pollutants	16-1	16-2	16-3					16-8				16-12	16-13			16-16					16-21	16-22	
Biological	17 Moulds	17-1	17-2	17-3					17-8				17-12			17-15	17-16	17-17	17-18	17-19	17-20	17-21	17-22	17-23
	18 Bacteria	18-1	18-2	18-3					18-8				18-12			18-15		18-17	18-18	18-19	18-20			
	19 MVOC								19-8				19-12			19-15		19-17	19-18	19-19				
	20 House dust	20-1	20-2	20-3					20-8			20-11					20-16	20-17	20-18		20-20			
Psychological, personal, other	21 Gender, working position			21-3																		21-21	21-22	21-23
	22 Social status																					22-21	22-22	22-23
	23 Other																					23-21	23-22	23-23

Fig. 4.2 Designed tool for decision-making process in the design of built environments Abbreviations: VOCs-volatile organic compounds, ETS-environmental tobacco smoke, MMMF- man-made mineral fibre, T_{ai}-air temperature, T_{surf}-surface temperature, RH_{ai}-relative humidity of indoor air, EM-electromagnetic fields, MVOC- microbes' volatile organic compounds

enables doing that and can be used as a tool for the decision-making process. It enables further upgrading according to new research findings.

BOX 4.5 Decision-making process in the design of built environments: case study

Step 1: Definition of the main problem, identifying hazards:
− Problem: appearance of mould (Fig. 4.3)
− Built environment: single room apartment, NE-oriented
− Infected active space: living room, bedroom
− Exposure population: 3 occupants
− Exposure time: 2 years, without noticeable health outcomes
− Duration: whole year, increase growth in October-March (temperate climate)
− Indicator: mould spots, draught environment
− Position, infected materials: final layers of constructional complexes, plaster; corners, behind furniture

Step 2. List of detected causes (building, system, user):
− Building: improper design of building envelope, inadequate composition of construction complexes (e.g., inadequate damp proof membrane, vapour barrier, thermal insulation, etc.), defects on intersections, geometric thermal bridges and construction thermal bridges (allows higher heat transfer than the surrounding thermal envelope), etc.
− system: inadequate ventilation, improper design of building envelope and system
− occupants' habits (cooking, indoor laundry drying)
− furniture position
− other possible causes are not present: irregularities in plumbing system, floods, etc.

Step 3. Definition of measures and step-by-step activities:
− specific goal: elimination of irregularities in construction complexes, systems, environment
− methods: measures of surface temperatures, material moisture content, indoor and outdoor environmental parameters; simulations of heat and moisture transfer before and after renovated construction complexes; characterization of mould species, concentration in air in special cases
− elimination of geometric and construction heat bridges with additional thermal insulation (upper part of the window, corner, etc.), installation of vapour barriers
− improved ventilation system in kitchen and bathroom
− elimination of irregularities in heating system
− education and training of all occupants (increased natural ventilation of all apartment, sock ventilation, drying laundry outdoors or in drying machine, use of ventilation devices in kitchen and bathroom etc.), increased distance between furniture position and wall

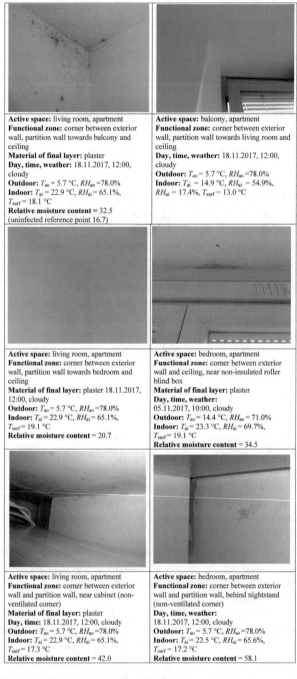

Fig. 4.3 Identified mouldy active spaces, functional zones, material and measured environmental parameters. Abbreviations: T_{ao} = outdoor air temperature (°C), RH_{ao} = relative air humidity of outdoor air (%), T_{ai} = indoor air temperature (°C), RH_{ai} = relative humidity of indoor air (%), T_{surf} = surface temperature of final layer (°C), relative moisture content measured on final layer

---

Step 4. Hazard calculation, comprehensive approach:
- interaction between parameters: definition of the consequences on other physical, chemical, biological health risk factors and their parameters: 1–17, 2–17, 3–17, 8–17, 12–17, 15–17, 17–17, 18–17, 19–17, 20–17
- optimal air temperature and relative air humidity levels according to user comfort and draught elimination

Step 5. Realization, efficiency evaluation:
- elimination of mould
- periodic monitoring of built environment, conditions and activities

---

With usage of the designed tool for decision-making process, similar activities, as it presented for mould (Fig. 4.3), can be performed for every detected problem in built environments (i.e., poor indoor air quality, thermal discomfort, etc.). Finally, the designed strategy includes holistic actions at the level of physical, chemical, biological, psychosocial, personal and other groups of risk factors and their interactive influences.

4.5   Short-Term and Long-Term Benefits of Holistic Design

It is expected that the implementation of design strategy will result in healthy and comfortable conditions, as well as increased productivity and decreased health costs with economic benefits. Moreover, such a holistic design of healthy built environments results in achieving overall efficiency of buildings, new or renovated ones. Construction or renovation leading to a healthy building results in minimized adverse health outcomes. This encourages a higher renovation rate that will bring large-scale benefits to individuals and society alike.

In addition to health, the environment, and the economy, the holistic design of healthy built environment renovations has several benefits (European Parliament 2016):

Environmental benefits: greenhouse gas emissions reduction, reduced usage of materials, energy savings,

Economic benefits: employment, GDP and public budgets, innovation, sectoral modernization, energy security, energy bill savings, increase in property value, tenant satisfaction,

Health benefits: reduction of energy poverty, productivity benefits, wellbeing, comfort benefits.

Up to today, many cost-benefit studies were performed to assess the financial benefits of performed activities for improving the quality of built environments. The potential financial benefits of improving indoor environments exceed costs by factors of 9 and 14 (Fisk 1999). For the US, Fisk and Rosenfeld (1997) estimated that potential annual savings and productivity gains ranged from $6 to $19 billion from reduced respiratory disease; $1–$4 billion from reduced allergies and asthma, $10–$20 billion from reduced symptoms of SBS, and $12–$125 billion from direct improvements in worker performance unrelated to health. Similar findings were recorded in the studies by Dutton et al. (2013) and Wargocki (2013).

Dutton et al. (2013) assessed the impact of a natural ventilation retrofit of 10% of

---

BOX 4.6 Cost-benefit analysis (CBA)

Cost-benefit analysis (CBA) offers a method of economic evaluation that values all benefits against all costs. The resulting cost-benefit ratio indicates whether or not the benefits outweigh the costs of an intervention and hence provides a decision-making tool with a broad societal perspective (WHO 2017).

California's office stock on the prevalence of SBS symptoms and associated costs; doing so would result in 22,000–56,000 fewer people reporting symptoms in a given week. Wargocki (2013) showed that crude estimates suggest that 2 million healthy life years can be saved in Europe by avoiding exposure to indoor air pollutants in non-industrial buildings. Healthy indoor air quality at work can increase people's productivity up to 10% (Wyon and Wargocki 2013). Similar estimates have been made for the U.S. as regards exposures to air pollutants in residential buildings. The potential annual savings and productivity gains have been estimated to be as high as $168 billion in the U.S. (1997 estimate as no newer data are available). A saving of $400 per employee per year (2000 estimate) was estimated due to reduced absenteeism being the result of improved indoor air quality. In Europe, the annual productivity benefits were estimated to be at the level of about €330 per worker (2000 estimate as no newer data are available) (Wargocki 2013). Recent studies have shown that costs of poor indoor environment for the employer, the building owner, and for society as a whole are often considerably higher than the cost of the energy used in the same building (EN 15251:2007).

Similar findings were made by:

Selkowitz, Energy Technologies Area (ETA), Lawrence Berkeley National Laboratory cautioned: "Very generally, if you look at costs in very round numbers, energy costs about $2 per square foot per year, and people cost about $200 per square foot" in an office building. So even a tiny improvement in productivity or sick time will pay off far more quickly than energy savings, he said (Washington Post 1999).

Temeljotov Salaj et al. (2017) highlighted the negative impacts of economic crises: "Economic crisis has impacts on workplace conditions, affects the satisfaction of employees and consequently occupational health. Implementing aspects of better workplace conditions introduces a better base of value for employees and employers", they concluded (Temeljotov Salaj et al. 2017, p. 2088).

In conclusion, well-designed buildings are those which are fit for their purpose (Lavin et al. 2006). Healthy buildings are more than that (Fig. 4.4).

The presented concept of healthy built environments with a design strategy is necessary for the future planning of healthy and comfortable buildings and is a basis for successful renovations. For this reason, it is essential to understand all benefits of such holistic approach as well as negative side-effects of current unilateral design

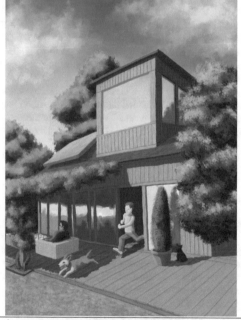

A healthy building is a component within healthy built environment and is the living or working environment in which all health risk factors are fully prevented, and optimal conditions for health and wellbeing of individual user are attained. Optimal conditions include stimulating and healing-oriented conditions, which result in fulfilment of specific needs for individual users and vulnerable ones.

Fig. 4.4 Concept of healthy built environments

that is currently in progress. Therefore, it is necessary to implement the strategy at the first step of design, at the planning stage.

Readers of this book acquire comprehensive knowledge and clear understanding of the health risk factors and their influences from various disciplines. In this way, it promotes multidisciplinary cooperation between various fields that is necessary for efficient control and prevention against negative health outcomes in built environments.

> All of us have responsibility to place human, as an individual and his values, in the front of design (Krašovec 2019).

References

Abdel-Hamid, M., Hakim, A. S., Elokda, E. E., & Mostafa, N. S. (2013). Prevalence and risk factors of sick building syndrome among office workers. *Journal of the Egyptian Public Health Association, 88,* 109–114. https://doi.org/10.1097/01.EPX.0000431629.28378.c0.

Assimakopoulos, V. D., & Helmis, C. G. (2004). On the study of a sick building: The case of Athens Air Traffic Control Tower. *Energy and Buildings, 36,* 15–22. https://doi.org/10.1016/S0378-7788(03)00043-4.

Azuma, K., Ikeda, K., Kagi, N., Yanagi, U., & Osawa, H. (2017). Physicochemical risk factors for building-related symptoms in air-conditioned office buildings: Ambient particles and combined exposure to indoor air pollutants. Science of the Total Environment 616–617:1649–1655. https://www.ncbi.nlm.nih.gov/pubmed/29070452. Retrieved December 3, 2018, from https://doi.org/10.1016/j.scitotenv.2017.10.147.

Bamai, Y. A., Araki, B. A., Kawai, T., Tsuboi, T., Saito, I., Yoshioka, E., et al. (2014). Associations of phthalate concentrations in floor dust and multi-surface dust with the interior materials in Japanese dwellings. *Science of the Total Environment, 468–469,* 147–157. https://doi.org/10.1016/j.scitotenv.2013.07.107.

Bamai, Y. A., Araki, A., Kawai, T., Tsuboi, T., Saito, I., Yoshioka, E., et al. (2016). Exposure to phthalates in house dust and associated allergies in children aged 6–12 years. *Environment International, 96,* 16–23. https://doi.org/10.1016/j.envint.2016.08.025.

Baričič, A., & Temeljotov Salaj, A. (2014). The impact of office workspace on the satisfaction of employees and their overall health - research presentation. *SlovMedJour, 83*(3), 217–231.

Bivolarova, M., Kierat, W., Zavrl, E., Popiolek, Z., & Melikov, A. (2017). Effect of airflow interaction in the breathing zone on exposure to bio-effluents. *Building and Environment, 125,* 216–226. https://doi.org/10.1016/j.buildenv.2017.08.043.

Blondel, A., & Plaisance, H. (2011). Screening of formaldehyde indoor sources and quantification of their emission using a passive sampler. *Building and Environment, 46,* 1284–1291. https://doi.org/10.1016/j.buildenv.2010.12.011.

Blount, B. C., Silva, M. J., Caudill, S. P., Needham, L. L., Pirkle, J. L., Sampson, E. J., et al. (2000). Levels of seven urinary phthalate metabolites in a human reference population. *Environmental Health Perspectives, 108,* 979–982. https://doi.org/10.1289/ehp.00108979.

Boardmann, B. (1991). *Fuel poverty: From cold homes to affordable warmth.* London: Belhaven Press.

Bornehag, C. G., Sundell, J., Weschler, C. J., Sigsgaard, T., Lundgren, B., Hasselgren, M., et al. (2004). The association between asthma and allergic symptoms in children and phthalates in house dust: a nested case–control study. *Environmental Health Perspectives, 112,* 1393–1397. https://doi.org/10.1289/ehp.7187.

BPIE. (2014). Buildings Performance Institute Europe. Alleviating fuel poverty in the EU investing in home renovation, a sustainable and inclusive solution. Retrieved November 9, 2018, from http://bpie.eu/wp-content/uploads/2015/10/Alleviating-fuel-poverty.pdf.

Burge, P. S. (2004). Sick building syndrome. *Occupational and Environmental Medicine, 61,* 185–190. https://doi.org/10.1136/oem.2003.008813.

Burt, T. (1996). Sick Building Syndrome: Acoustic Aspects. *Indoor and Built Environment, 5*(1), 44–59. http://smithvilleturbinesoppositionparty.ca/news/wp-content/uploads/2015/03/Indoor-and-Built-Environment-1996-Burt-44-59.pdf. Retrieved December 3, 2018, from http://dx.doi.org/10.1177/1420326X9600500107.

CDC. (2015). The National Institute for Occupational Safety and Health (NIOSH) Indoor Environmental Quality. Chemicals and Odors. Retrieved December 3, 2017, from https://www.cdc.gov/niosh/topics/indoorenv/chemicalsodors.html.

Chen, Z., Shi, J., Shen, X., Ma, Q., & Xu, B. (2016). Study on formaldehyde emissions from porous building material under non-isothermal conditions. *Applied Thermal Engineering, 101,* 165–172. https://doi.org/10.1016/j.applthermaleng.2016.02.134.

Choi, H., Schmidbauer, N., & Bornehag, C.-G. (2017). Volatile organic compounds of possible microbial origin and their risks on childhood asthma and allergies within damp homes. *Environment International, 98,* 143–151. https://doi.org/10.1016/j.envint.2016.10.028.

Clausen, P., Liu, Z., Kofoed-Sørensen, V., Little, J., & Wolkoff, P. (2012). Influence of temperature on the emission of di-(2-ethylhexyl) phthalate (DEHP) from PVC flooring in the emission cell FLEC. *Environmental Science and Technology, 17*(46), 909–915. https://doi.org/10.1021/es2035625.

Costa, M., & Brickus, L. (2000). Effects of ventilation systems on prevalence of symptoms associated with sick buildings in Brazilian commercial establishments. *Archives of Environmental Health, 55,* 279–283. https://doi.org/10.1080/00039890009603419.

Delfino, R. J. (2002). Epidemiologic evidence for asthma and exposure to air toxics: linkages between occupational, indoor, and community air pollution research. *Environmental Health Perspectives, 110*(4), 573–589. https://doi.org/10.1289/ehp.02110s4573.

Douwes, J., Thorne, P., Pearce, N., & Heederik, D. (2003). Bioaerosol health effects and exposure assessment: Progress and prospects. *Annals of Occupational Hygiene, 47*(3), 187–200. https://doi.org/10.1093/annhyg/meg032.

Dovjak, M., & Kristl, Ž. (2011). Health concerns of PVC materials in the built environment. *International Journal Sanitary Engineering Research, 5,* 4–26.

Dutton, S. M., Banks, D., Brunswick, S. L., & Fisk, W. J. (2013). Health and economic implications of natural ventilation in California offices. *Building and Environment, 67,* 34–45. https://doi.org/10.1016/j.buildenv.2013.05.002.

ECA. (1989). Indoor air quality & its impact on man. COST Project 613. Environment and Quality of Life Report No. 4. Sick Building Syndrome. A Practical Guide. In. Luxembourg.: Commission of the European Communities. Directorate General for Science. Research and Development. Joint Research Centre - Institute for the Environment. Commission of the European Communities, ECA.

Ecofys. (2017). The relation between quality of dwelling, socio-economic status and health in EU28 and its Member States. Scientific report as input for Healthy Homes, Barometer 2017, Hermelink A, Ashok J. Retrieved December 3, 2018, from http://www.ecofys.com/files/files/ecofys-2017-relation-between-quality-of-dwelling-and-health-final.pdf.

Eder, W., Ege, M. J., & von Mutius, E. (2006). The asthma epidemic. *New England Journal of Medicine, 355,* 2226–2235. https://doi.org/10.1056/NEJMra054308.

EN. (15251:2007). Indoor environmental input parameters for design and assessment of energy performance of buildings addressing indoor air quality, thermal environment, lighting and acoustics.

Engvall, K. (2000). Development of a multiple regression model to identify multi-family residential buildings with a high prevalence of sick building syndrome (SBS). *Indoor Air, 10,* 101–110. https://doi.org/10.1034/j.1600-0668.2000.010002101.x.

EPA. (2017). VOC. Retrieved December 3, 2018, from https://www.epa.gov/indoor-air-quality-iaq/volatile-organic-compounds-impact-indoor-air-quality.

EPEE. (2017). European fuel Poverty and Energy Efficiency (EPEE). Epee Project. Retrieved December 3, 2018, from https://ec.europa.eu/energy/intelligent/projects/en/projects/epee.

Eurostat. (2017). Housing conditions. Retrieved December 3, 2018, from http://ec.europa.eu/eurostat/statistics-explained/index.php/Housing_conditions.

European Parliament. (2016). Directorate general for internal policies policy department A: Economic and scientific policy. In I. Artola, K. Rademaekers, R. Williams, J. Yearwood (Eds.), *Boosting building renovation: What potential and value for Europe?* Retrieved December 3, 2018, from http://www.europarl.europa.eu/RegData/etudes/STUD/2016/587326/IPOL_STU (2016)587326_EN.pdf.

Fiedler, K., Schütz, E., Geh, S. (2001). Detection of microbial volatile organic compounds (MVOCs) produced by moulds on various materials. *International Journal of Hygiene and Environmental Health, 204*(2–3), 111–121. https://ac.els-cdn.com/S1438463904700826/1-s2. 0-S1438463904700826-main.pdf?_tid=1b14e6dc-d4f9-11e7-a4e2-00000aab0f01&acdnat= 1511955382_ed059f335714e49946d64694b22b87e3. Retrieved December 3, 2017, from. http://dx.doi.org/10.1078/1438-4639-00094.

Findeis, H., & Peters, E. (2004). Disturbing effects of low frequency sound immissions and vibrations in residential buildings. *Noise Health, 6*(23), 29–35. Retrieved December 3, 2017 from https://www.ncbi.nlm.nih.gov/pubmed/15273022.

Fisk, W. J. (1999). Estimates of potential nationwide productivity and health benefits from better indoor environments: An update. In: J. Spengler, J. Samet, & J. McCarthy (2001) *Indoor air quality handbook* McGraw Hill: McGraw-Hill Education. Retrieved December 3, 2018 from https://www.accessengineeringlibrary.com/browse/indoor-air-quality-handbook.

Fisk, W. J. & Rosenfeld, A. H. (1997). Estimates of improved productivity and health from better indoor environments. *Indoor Air 7*(3), 158–172. https://indoor.lbl.gov/publications/estimates-improved-productivity-and. Retrieved December 3, 2017 from http://dx.doi.org/10.1111/j. 1600-0668.1997.t01-1-00002.x.

Frontczak, M., & Wargocki, P. (2011). Literature survey on how different factors influence human comfort in indoor environments. *Building and Environment, 46,* 922–937. https://doi.org/10. 1016/j.buildenv.2010.10.021.

Gustafsson, Å., Krais, A. M., Gorzsás, A., Lundh, T., & Gerde, P. (2018) Isolation and characterization of a respirable particle fraction from residential house-dust. *Environmental Research, 161,* 284–290. http://www.sciencedirect.com/science/article/pii/ S0013935117316717 Retrieved December 3, 2017 from http://dx.doi.org/10.1016/j.envres. 2017.10.049.

Grant, C., Hunter, C. A., Flannigan, B., & Bravery, A. F. (1989). The moisture requirements of moulds isolated from domestic dwellings. *International Biodeterioration, 25*(4), 259–284. https://doi.org/10.1016/0265-3036(89)90002-X.

Haghighat, F., & De Bellis, L. (1998). Material emission rates: literature review, and the impact of indoor air temperature and relative humidity. *Building and Environment, 33,* 261–277. https:// doi.org/10.1016/S0360-1323(97)00060-7.

Heudorf, U., Mersch-Sundermann, V., & Angerer, J. (2007). Phthalates: toxicology and exposure. *International Journal of Hygiene and Environmental Health, 210,* 623–634. https://doi.org/10. 1016/j.ijheh.2007.07.011.

Hodgson, M., Permar, E., Squire, G., Allera, C. W., & Parkinson, D. K. (1987) Vibrations as a cause of "tight-building syndrome" symptoms. *ibid, 2,* 449–453.

Hodgson, A. T. (2000). Volatile organic compound concentrations and emission rates in new manufactured and site-built houses. *Indoor Air, 10,* 178–192. https://doi.org/10.1034/j.1600-0668.2000.010003178.x.

Huang, S., Xiong, J., & Zhang, Y. (2015). The impact of relative humidity on the emission behaviour of formaldehyde in building materials. *Procedia Engineering, 121,* 59–66. https://doi.org/10.1016/j.proeng.2015.08.1019.

Huang, C., Liu, W., Cai, J., Wang, X., Zou, Z., & Sun, C. (2017). Household formaldehyde exposure and its associations with dwelling characteristics, lifestyle behaviours, and childhood health outcomes in Shanghai, China. *Building and Environment, 125,* 143–152. https://doi.org/10.1016/j.buildenv.2017.08.042.

Jaakkola, J., Heinonen, O., & Seppänen, O. (1989). Sick building syndrome, sensation of dryness and thermal comfort in relation to room temperature in an office building: Need for individual control of temperature. *Environment International 15,* 163–168. Retrieved December 3, 2017 from http://dx.doi.org/10.1016/0160-4120(89)90022-6.

Jaakkola, J., Oie, L., Nafstad, P., Botten, G., Samuelsen, S. O., & Magnus, P. (1999). Surface materials in the home and development of bronchial obstruction in young children in Oslo, Norway. *American Journal of Public Health, 84*(2), 188–192. https://doi.org/10.2105/AJPH.89.2.188.

Järnström, H., Saarela, K., Kalliokoski, P., & Pasanenc, A.-L. (2006). Reference values for indoor air pollutant concentrations in new, residential buildings in Finland. *Atmospheric Environment, 40,* 7178–7191. https://doi.org/10.1016/j.atmosenv.2006.06.021.

Jiang, C., Li, D., Zhang, P., Li, J., Wang, J., & Yu, J. (2017). Formaldehyde and volatile organic compound (VOC) emissions from particleboard: Identification of odorous compounds and effects of heat treatment. *Building and Environment, 117,* 118–126. https://doi.org/10.1016/j.buildenv.2017.03.004.

Johansson, P., Bok, G., & Ekstrand-Tobin, A. (2013). The effect of cyclic moisture and temperature on mould growth on wood compared to steady state conditions. *Building and Environment, 65,* 178–184. https://doi.org/10.1016/j.buildenv.2013.04.004.

Kajiwara, N., & Takigami, H. (2016). Particle size distribution of brominated flame retardants in house dust from Japan. *Emerging Contaminants, 2*(2), 109–117. https://doi.org/10.1016/j.emcon.2016.03.005.

Kaminsky, D. A. (2012). What does airway resistance tell us about lung function? *Respiratory Care, 57*(1), 85–96. https://doi.org/10.4187/respcare.01411.

Kim, S. S., Kang, D. H., Choi, D. H., Yeo, M. S., & Kim, W. K. (2012). VOC emission from building materials in residential buildings with radiant floor heating systems. *Aerosol and Air Quality Research, 12,* 1398–1408. https://doi.org/10.4209/aaqr.2011.11.0222.

Kishi, R., Araki, A., Saitoh, I., Shibata, E., Morimoto, K., Nakayama, K., et al. (2012). Phthalate in house dust and its relation to sick building syndrome and allergic symptoms. In *30th International Congress on Occupational Health organized in Cancun from March 18th to March 23rd, 2012,* Mexico.

Kontonasiou, E., Atanasiu, B., & Mariottini, F. (2015). Fuel poverty mitigation through energy efficiency in buildings. BPIE EU, Buildings Performance Institute Europe, Bruxelles. Retrieved December 3, 2018 from http://bpie.eu/wp-content/uploads/2015/10/BPIEposter-Fuel-Poverty20151.pdf.

Krašovec, J. (2019). Human values of an individual in space and time. Vrednote človeka kot osebnega bitja v prostoru in času. In: M. Dovjak, J. Krašovec (Eds.), *Role and meaning of individual in the process of building construction.* Invited lecture. Vloga in pomen posameznika v procesu graditve stavb. Invited lecture. Dvorana Slovenske matice, Ljubljana, 26.02.2019. Retrieved Februay 28, 2019, from http://www.slovenska-matica.si/events/predavanje-vloga-pomen-posameznika-v-procesu-graditve-stavb/.

Lappalainen, V., Sohlberg, E., Järnström, H., Laamanen, J., Viitanen, H., & Pasanen, P. (2015). IAQ simulator tests: VOC emissions from hidden mould growth. *Energy Procedia, 78,* 1212–1217. https://doi.org/10.1016/j.egypro.2015.11.187.

Lavin, T., Higgins, C., Metcalfe, O., & Jordan, A. (2006). Health impacts of the built environment a review. Institute of Public Health in Ireland, July 2006. Retrieved December 3, 2018, from https://www.publichealth.ie/files/file/Health_Impacts_of_the_Built_Environment_A_Review.pdf.

Law, A. K. Y., Chau, C. K., & Chan, G. Y. S. (2001). Characteristics of bioaerosol profile in office buildings in Hong Kong. *Building and Environment, 36*(4), 527–541. https://doi.org/10.1016/S0360-1323(00)00020-2.

Lu, C. Y., Ma, Y. C., Lin, J. M., Li, C. Y., Lin, R. S., & Sung, F. C. (2007). Oxidative stress associated with indoor air pollution and sick building syndrome-related symptoms among office workers in Taiwan. *Inhalation Toxicology, 19,* 57–65. https://doi.org/10.1080/08958370600985859.

Lu, C., Deng, Q., Li, Y., Sundell, J., & Norbäck, D. (2016). Outdoor air pollution, meteorological conditions and indoor factors in dwellings in relation to sick building syndrome (SBS) among adults in China. *Science of the Total Environment* 560–561, 186–196. http://www.sciencedirect.com/science/article/pii/S0048969716307148. Retrieved December 3, 2017, from http://dx.doi.org/10.1016/j.scitotenv.2016.04.033.

Malkin, J. (2008). *A visual reference for evidence-based design.* Concord, CA, USA: Center for Health Design.

Metin Özcan, K., Gülay, E., & Üçdoğruk, S. (2013). Economic and demographic determinants of household energy use in Turkey. *Energy Policy, 60,* 550–557. https://doi.org/10.1016/j.enpol.2013.05.046.

Mizoue, T., Reijula, K., & Andersson, K. (2001). Environmental tobacco smoke exposure and overtime work as risk factors for sick building syndrome in Japan. *American Journal of Epidemiology, 154,* 803–808. https://doi.org/10.1093/aje/154.9.803.

Nakaoka, H., Todaka, E., Seto, H., Saito, I., Hanazato, M., Watanabe, M., et al. (2014). Correlating the symptoms of sick-building syndrome to indoor VOCs concentration levels and odour. *Indoor and Built Environment, 23,* 804–813. https://doi.org/10.1177/1420326X13500975.

Nimmermark, S., & Gustafsson, G. (2005). Influence of temperature, humidity, and ventilation rate on the release of odour and ammonia in a floor housing system for laying hens. *Agricultural Engineering International, VII* 15.

NIPH. (2012). *Guidelines for reducing the risk of Legionella growth.* Ljubljana: NIPH.

Omrani, S., Garcia-Hansen, V., Capra, B. R., & Drogemuller, R. (2017). Effect of natural ventilation mode on thermal comfort and ventilation performance: Full-scale measurement. *Energy Buildings, 156,* 1–16. http://dx.doi.org/10.1016/j.enbuild.2017.09.061.

Ooi, P., & Goh, K. (1997). Sick building syndrome: an emerging stress-related disorder? *International Journal of Epidemiology, 26,* 1243–1249. https://doi.org/10.1093/ije/26.6.1243.

Park, J. H., Spiegelman, D. L., Gold, D. R., Burge, H. A., & Milton, D. K. (2001). Predictors of airborne endotoxin in the home. *Environmental Health Perspectives, 109*(8), 859–864. https://doi.org/10.1289/ehp.01109859.

Paustenbach, D. J. (2002). *Human and ecological risk assessment: Theory and pactice* (1st ed.). D. J. Paustenbach, &W. K. Reilly (Foreword). John Wiley and Sons, New York.

Peat, J., Dickerson, J., & Li, J. (1998). Effects of damp and mould in the home on respiratory health: a review of the literature. *Allergy, 53,* 120–128. https://doi.org/10.1111/j.1398-9995.1998.tb03859.x.

Prussin, A. J., Schwake, O. D., & Marr, L. C. (2017). Ten questions concerning the aerosolization and transmission of Legionella in the built environment. *Building and Environment, 123,* 684–695. https://doi.org/10.1016/j.buildenv.2017.06.024.

Recek, P. (2017). *The quality of indoor environment in association with socio-economic indicators.* Pilot Study: Faculty of Health Sciences, University of Ljubljana, Ljubljana.

Recek, P., Kump, T., & Dovjak, M. (2019). Indoor environmental quality in relation to socioeconomic indicators in Slovenian households. *Journal of Housing and the Built Environment.* https://doi.org/10.1007/s10901-019-09659-x.

Redlich, C. A., Sparer, J., & Cullen, M. R. (1997). Sick-building syndrome. *The Lancet, 349,* 1013–1016. https://doi.org/10.1016/S0140-6736(96)07220-0.

Sahlberg, B., Gunnbjörnsdottir, M., Soon, A., Jogi, R., Gislason, T., Wieslander, G., et al. (2013). Airborne molds and bacteria, microbial volatile organic compounds (MVOC), plasticizers and formaldehyde in dwellings in three North European cities in relation to sick building syndrome (SBS). *Science of the Total Environment, 444,* 433–440. https://doi.org/10.1016/j.scitotenv.2012.10.114.

Sakai, K., Norbäck, D., Mi, Y., Shibata, E., Kamijima, M., Yamada, T., et al. (2004). A comparison of indoor air pollutants in Japan and Sweden: formaldehyde, nitrogen dioxide, and chlorinated volatile organic compounds. *Environmental Research, 94,* 75–85. https://doi.org/10.1016/S0013-9351(03)00140-3.

Salthammer, T., Mentese, S., & Marutzky, R. (2010). Formaldehyde in the indoor environment. *Chemical Reviews, 110,* 2536–2572. https://doi.org/10.1021/cr800399g.

Salimifard, P., Rim, D., Gomes, C., Kremer, P., & Freihaut, J. D. (2017). Resuspension of biological particles from indoor surfaces: Effects of humidity and air swirl. *Science of the Total Environment, 583,* 241–247. https://doi.org/10.1016/j.scitotenv.2017.01.058.

Santamouris, M., Kapsis, K., Korres, D., Livada, I., Pavlou, C., & Assimakopoulos, M. N. (2007). On the relation between the energy and social characteristics of the residential sector. *Energy Build 39*(8), 893–905. Retrieved December 3, 2018, from http://dx.doi.org/10.1016/j.enbuild.2006.11.001.

Sautour, M., Soares Mansur, C., Divies, C., Bensoussan, M., & Dantigny, P. (2002). Comparison of the effects of temperature and water activity on growth rate of food spoilage moulds. *Journal of Industrial Microbiology & Biotechnology, 28,* 311–315. https://doi.org/10.1038/sj.jim.7000248.

Schwartz, S. (2008). Linking noise and vibration to sick building syndrome in office buildings 2008. Air & Waste Management Association. Retrieved December 3, 2018, from http://sandischwartz.com/wp-content/uploads/2015/07/EM_Magazine_final_printed_article.pdf.

Sekulska, M., Piotraszewska-Pająk, A., Szyszka, A., Nowicki, M., & Filipiak, M. (2007). Microbiological quality of indoor air in university rooms. *Polish Journal of Environmental Studies, 16*(4), 623–632.

Seppänen, O., Fisk, W., & Mendell, M. (1999). Association of ventilation rates and CO_2 concentrations with health and other responses in commercial and industrial buildings. *Indoor Air, 9,* 226–252. https://doi.org/10.1111/j.1600-0668.1999.00003.x.

Seppänen, O., & Fisk, W. (2002). Association of ventilation system type with SBS symptoms in office workers. *Indoor Air, 12,* 98–112. https://doi.org/10.1034/j.1600-0668.2002.01111.x.

Shan, X., Zhou, J., Chang, V. W.-C., & Yan, E.-H. (2016) Comparing mixing and displacement ventilation in tutorial rooms: Students' thermal comfort, sick building syndromes, and short-term performance. *Building and Environment, 102,* 128–137. http://dx.doi.org/10.1016/j.buildenv.2016.03.025.

Sheehan, P., Singhal, A., Bogen, K. T., MacIntosh, D., Kalmes, R. M., & McCarthy, J. (2017). Potential exposure and cancer risk from formaldehyde emissions from installed Chinese manufactured laminate flooring. *Risk Analysis, 38*(6), 1128–1142. https://doi.org/10.1111/risa.12926.

Sierra-Vargas, M. P., & Teran, L. M. (2012). Air pollution: Impact and prevention. *Respirology, 17*(7), 1031–1038.

Skov, P., Valbjorn, O., & Pedersen, B. V. (1990). Influence of indoor climate on the sick building syndrome in an office environment. *Scandinavian Journal of Work, Environment & Health, 16* (5), 363–371.

Smallwood, J. (2018). 7: Reducing static electricity in carpets. In *Advances in carpet manufacture* (2nd ed., pp. 135–162). The textile institute book series https://doi.org/10.1016/B978-0-08-101131-7.00008-3.

Subedi, B., Sullivan, K. D., & Dhungana, B. (2017). Phthalate and non-phthalate plasticizers in indoor dust from childcare facilities, salons, and homes across the USA. *Environmental Pollution, 230,* 701–708. https://doi.org/10.1016/j.envpol.2017.07.028.

Sun, C., Huang, C., Liu, W., Zou, Z., Hu, Y., & Shen, L. (2017). Home dampness-related exposures increase the risk of common colds among preschool children in Shanghai, China: Modified by household ventilation. *Building and Environment, 124,* 31–41. https://doi.org/10.1016/j.buildenv.2017.07.033.

Šarić, M., Kulcar, Z., Zorica, M., & Gelić, I. (1976). Malignant tumors of the liver and lungs in an area with a PVC industry. *Environmental Health Perspectives, 17,* 189–192. https://doi.org/10.1289/ehp.7617189.

Šestan, P., Kristl, Ž., & Dovjak, M. (2013). Formaldehyde in the built environment and its potential impact on human health. *Gradbeni vestnik, 62,* 191–203.

Takeuchi, S., Kojima, H., Saito, I., Jin, K., Kobayashi, S., Tanaka-Kagawa, T., et al. (2014). Detection of 34 plasticizers and 25 flame retardants in indoor air from houses in Sapporo, Japan. *Science of the Total Environment, 491–492,* 28–33. https://doi.org/10.1016/j.scitotenv. 2014.04.011.

Takigawa, T., Saijo, Y., Morimoto, K., Nakayama, K., Shibata, E., Tanaka, M., et al. (2012). A longitudinal study of aldehydes and volatile organic compounds associated with subjective symptoms related to sick building syndrome in new dwellings in Japan. *Science of the Total Environment, 417–418,* 61–67. https://doi.org/10.1016/j.scitotenv.2011.12.060.

Teeuw, K., Vandenbroucke-Grauls, C., & Verhoef, J. (1994). Airborne gram-negative bacteria and endotoxin in sick building syndrome. A study in Dutch governmental office buildings. *Archives of Internal Medicine, 154,* 2339–2345. https://doi.org/10.1001/archinte.154.20.2339.

Temeljotov Salaj, A., Maamari, B., Baričič, A., & Lohne, J. (2015). The influence of workplace on overall health in Slovenia and Lebanon-empirical research. *HealthMed, 9*(7), 281–300.

Temeljotov Salaj, A., Baričič, A., & Maamari, B. (2017). How the economic crisis affects workplace conditions and occupational health. *Journal of Construction Project Management and Innovation, 7*(2), 2088–2103.

Velux. (2016). The healthy homes barometer 2016. Retrieved December 3, 2018, from http:// www.velux.com/article/2016/energy-renovation-resonates-with-european-home-owners.

Velux Group. (2017). Healthy homes barometer 2017. Retrieved December 3, 2018, from http:// velcdn.azureedge.net/ ∼ /media/com/health/healthy-home-barometer/507505-01% 20barometer_2017.pdf.

Verreault, D., Moineau, S., & Duchaine, C. (2008). Methods for sampling of airborne viruses. *Microbiology and Molecular Biology Reviews, 72*(3), 413–444. https://doi.org/10.1128/ MMBR.00002-08.

Wang, J., Li, B., Yang, Q., Yu, W., Wang, H., Norback, D., et al. (2013). Odors and sensations of humidity and dryness in relation to sick building syndrome and home environment in Chongqing, China. *PLoS One, 8,* e72385 http://journals.plos.org/plosone/article?id=10.1371/ journal.pone.0072385. Retrieved December 3, 2017, from http://dx.doi.org/10.1371/journal. pone.0072385.

Wargocki, P. (2013). Productivity and health effects of high indoor air quality. In *Reference module in earth systems and environmental sciences.* https://www.sciencedirect.com/science/ article/pii/B978012409548901993X. Retrieved December 3, 2018, from http://dx.doi.org/10. 1016/B978-0-12-409548-9.01993-X.

Washington Post. (1999). Daylighting and productivity-CEC PIER. Study says natural classroom lighting can aid achievement. By Cooper KJ. Washington Post Staff Writer Washington Post, Friday, November 26, 1999, Page A14. Retrieved December 3, 2018, from http://h-m-g.com/ projects/daylighting/publicity%20daylighting.htm.

WHECA. (2000). Warm homes and energy conservation act 2000. Retrieved December 3, 2018, from https://www.legislation.gov.uk/ukpga/2000/31/contents.

WHO. (2004). *Children's health and the environment.* Geneva: World Health Organization.

WHO. (2012). Environmental health inequalities in Europe. Retrieved December 3, 2018, from http://www.euro.who.int/__data/assets/pdf_file/0010/157969/e96194.pdf?ua=1.

WHO. (2017). Indoor air pollution. Cost-benefit analysis of interventions. Retrieved December 3, 2017, from http://www.who.int/indoorair/interventions/cost_benefit/en/.

Weichenthal, S., Dufresne, A., & Infante-Rivard, C. (2007). Indoor ultrafine particles and childhood asthma: Exploring a potential public health concern. *Indoor Air, 17,* 81–91. https:// doi.org/10.1111/j.1600-0668.2006.00446.x.

Wieslander, G., Norback, D., & Venge, P. (2007). Changes of symptoms, tear film stability and eosinophilic cationic protein in nasal lavage fluid after re-exposure to a damp office building with a history of flooding. *Indoor Air, 17,* 19–27. https://doi.org/10.1111/j.1600-0668.2006. 00441.x.

Wyon, D. F., & Wargocki, P. (2013). Effects of indoor environment on performance. *ASHRAE Journal 46*–50. Retrieved November 10, 2017, from http://www.rehva.eu/fileadmin/REHVA_Journal/REHVA_Journal_2013/RJ_issue_4/p.6/06-10-RJ1304_web.pdf.

Xu, J., & Zhang, J. S. (2011). An experimental study of relative humidity effect on VOCs effective diffusion coefficient and partition coefficient in a porous medium. *Building and Environment, 46*(9), 1785–1796. https://doi.org/10.1016/j.buildenv.2011.02.007.

Xu, Y., Cohen Hubal, E., & Little, J. (2009). Predicting residential exposure to phthalate plasticizer emitted from vinyl flooring: a mechanistic analysis. *Environmental Science and Technology, 43,* 2374–2380. https://doi.org/10.1021/es801354f.

Yassi, A., Kjellstrom, T., de Kok, T., & Guidotti, T. (2001). Basic environmental health: Oxford University Press, Inc.

Yassin, M., & Almouqatea, S. (2010). Assessment of airborne bacteria and fungi in an indoor and outdoor environment. *International Journal of Environmental Science and Technology, 7*(3), 535–544. https://doi.org/10.1007/BF03326162.

Yun, G. Y., & Steemers, K. (2011). Behavioural, physical and socio-economic factors in household cooling energy consumption. *Applied Energy, 88*(6), 2191–2200. https://doi.org/10.1016/j.apenergy.2011.01.010.

Zak, J. C., & Wildman, H. G. (2004) 14-Fungi in stressful environments. In *Biodiversity of fungi* (pp. 303–315). Burlington: Academic Press.

Zhu, L., Deng, B., & Guo, Y. (2013). A unified model for VOCs emission/sorption from/on building materials with and without ventilation. *International Journal of Heat and Mass Transfer, 67,* 734–740. http://www.sciencedirect.com/science/article/pii/S001793101300762X. Retrieved December 3, 2018, from http://dx.doi.org/10.1016/j.ijheatmasstransfer.2013.08.092.

Zhang, Y., Luo, X., Wang, X., Qian, K., & Zhao, R. (2007). Influence of temperature on formaldehyde emission parameters of dry building materials. *Atmospheric Environment, 41* (15), 3203–3216. https://doi.org/10.1016/j.atmosenv.2006.10.081.

Zhang, X., Sahlberg, B., Wieslander, G., Janson, C., Gislason, T., & Norback, D. (2012). Dampness and moulds in workplace buildings: Associations with incidence and remission of sick building syndrome (SBS) and biomarkers of inflammation in a 10 year follow-up study. *Science of the total environment, 430,* 75–81.

Zinn, T. W., Cline, D., & Lehmann, W. F. (1990). Long-term study of formaldehyde emission decay from particleboard. *Forest Products Journal, 40*(6), 15–18.

Index

A

Absenteeism, 69, 93, 146
Acclimatization, 49, 52
Active space, 11, 14
Active zone, 11
Adjusted Odds Ratio (AOR), 104
Adverse health effects, 32, 60, 68–70, 73, 84, 86, 87, 90, 93, 94, 97–99, 124, 126, 136
Adverse health outcomes, 145
Aetiology, 61
Age, 32, 33, 49, 52, 54, 66, 70, 72, 73, 85, 94, 95, 99, 108, 110, 126, 134, 136, 137, 138
Air-conditioned offices, 92, 129
Air humidity, 14, 16, 18, 29, 51, 64, 73, 89, 90, 97, 100, 123, 124, 132, 142, 145
Air quality, 8, 11, 12, 29–32, 47, 49, 56, 58, 60, 64, 66, 91, 95, 97, 101, 106, 125, 127, 136, 138, 146
Air temperature, 11, 14–18, 30, 32, 51, 53, 73, 89, 90, 123, 127–129, 132, 138, 141, 142, 144, 145
Air velocity, 51, 89, 123, 127, 128
Aldehydes, 100, 129
Allergens, 61, 97, 104, 131
Anthropogenic activities, 3
Asbestos, 60, 66, 96

B

Bacteria, 88, 105, 132
Basic requirements, 12, 22
Bioclimatic design, 5, 8, 10
Bioclimatic endowment, 9

Biological risk factors, 87
Building airtightness, vii
Building characteristics, 88, 110, 138, 139
Building dampness, 63, 64, 68, 132
Building energy use, 1, 30
Building envelope(/-s), vii, 10, 26, 27, 90, 123
Building-Related Illness (BRI), 60–62, 104, 131
Building users, vii, 47
Built environments(/-s), 1–4, 7, 8, 13, 14, 24, 25, 27, 32, 33, 43, 44, 47, 48, 52, 54, 60, 63, 69, 70, 73, 74, 83–89, 92, 93, 96, 103, 107–110, 121, 122, 127, 134, 140, 143–145, 147, 148

C

Cause-effect relationship, viii
Chemical risk factors, 87
Children, 8, 13, 14, 26, 32, 33, 59, 63, 64, 66, 68, 71, 93, 98–100, 106, 126, 129, 131, 136, 138
Circadian rhythms, 32, 33
Cleaning sprays, 97
Climate, 7–9, 22–24, 26, 33, 73, 90, 108, 109, 137, 143
Climate change, 8, 65
Clothing, 14, 51, 89, 96, 99, 123, 138
CO_2, 20, 23, 29, 30, 69, 101, 102, 109, 127, 130, 137
CO_2 concentrations, 29, 102
Communication, 20, 34, 67, 88, 122
Confidence Interval (CI), 106, 133
Construction product, 21

© The Author(s) 2019
M. Dovjak and A. Kukec, *Creating Healthy and Sustainable Buildings*, https://doi.org/10.1007/978-3-030-19412-3

157

Construction works, 12, 21–23
Cost-Benefit Analysis (CBA), 146

D
Dampness, 90, 103, 120, 129
Daylight (/-ing), 12, 27, 30, 33, 46, 47, 49, 58,
        60, 63, 68–70, 86, 88, 89, 92, 93
Decision-making, 140, 141, 143–145
Design, 1, 2, 4–12, 14, 15, 19, 21, 25–30,
        32–35, 46–49, 54, 57, 58, 60, 64, 73, 85,
        88, 89, 95–97, 102, 108, 121, 123, 124,
        127, 138, 140, 141, 143–145, 147
Design ventilation rates, 30
Determinants of health, 24, 83, 84
Diagnosis, 61
Disinfection, 11, 12, 28, 88
Dose-response relationship, 107
Duration, 61, 143
Dwellings, vii, 26, 31, 104–107, 110, 128, 135,
        137, 139

E
Eco-friendly building, viii, 43, 54, 57
Elderly, 8, 9, 13, 26, 33, 34, 52, 59, 65, 71, 72,
        135, 136
Electromagnetic fields, 88, 123
Energy efficiency, 10, 20, 23, 24, 26, 27, 29,
        34, 58, 70, 136
Energy inefficient, vii
Energy performance, vii
Engineering and public health perspectives, 1
Environmental benefits, 145
Environmental factors, 32, 45, 54, 61, 85, 107,
        128, 134
Environmental hazard, 60
Environmental health inequalities, 135
Environmental health risk factors, vii
Environmental parameters, 48, 88, 89
Environmental protection, 1
Environmental public health, 3, 45, 60
Environmental stressors, 32
Environmental tobacco smoke, 60, 66, 88, 94,
        96, 100, 101, 125, 139, 144
Ergonomics, 12, 46, 49, 53, 88, 95, 96
Evidence based design approach, 141
Exposure dose, 60, 87
Exposure time, 60, 87, 107
External risk factors, 72

F
Firmitas, 7
Formaldehyde, 29, 30, 86, 88, 95–98, 102, 103,
        106, 125, 127, 128, 138, 141
Fuel poverty, 134, 135

Functional zone, 12

G
Gender, 49, 51, 52, 72, 84, 88, 108, 134
Geopathic stress, 110
Geopathogenic zones, 88, 110
Green building, viii, 43, 54, 57

H
Hazardous substances, 66
Health, 3, 12, 16, 19, 24, 25, 30, 43, 45, 48, 54,
        56, 59, 60, 63, 66, 72, 73, 84–87, 97,
        101, 103, 122, 141, 145
Health benefits, 145
Health characteristics, 108
Health determinants, 44, 47, 108, 109
Health effects, 60
Health Risk Assessment (HRA), 86, 87
Health risk parameters, vii
Health status, 16, 49, 52, 58, 63, 70, 88, 134
Healthy and comfortable built environments,
        vii
Healthy and comfortable conditions, 24, 145
Healthy and sustainable buildings, viii, 1, 58
Healthy buildings (/-s), viii, 45–47, 49, 50, 58,
        63, 145
Healthy built environment, 9, 47, 141, 145
Heat-related mortality, 7, 65
Helplessness, 88, 108
Hidden olfs, 100
Hippodamian plan, 1
Holistic approach, 147
Homeostasis, 48
House dust, 88, 103, 107, 130, 131
Household products, 88, 96, 97, 99, 100,
        124–127
Human-made environment, 3
Human-made space, 1
Human needs, 2, 48, 49
Human performance, 32
Humidifiers, 97, 133
HVAC systems, 19, 27, 52, 91, 130, 131

I
Identification, viii, 74, 83, 86, 121, 122, 137,
        140
Inadequate housing conditions, 31
Inadequate living and working conditions, 26
Inadequate ventilation, 91
Individual characteristics, 44, 51, 60, 83, 87,
        108
Individual needs and demands, 4
Individual perceptions, 52
Indoor built environments, vii

Indoor environmental quality, vii, 29, 50, 58, 60, 92, 100, 134, 135
Industrialization, 3
Insect, 88
Insecticides (/-s), 88, 100, 110, 126
Internal risk factors, 72
Ions, 88, 123

L
Legionella spp., 28
Legislation, vii, 1, 5, 20, 23, 25, 26, 28–30, 125
Life cycles, viii
Location, viii, 5, 7–10, 23, 59, 63, 65, 88, 97, 110, 123
Location endowments, 5
Loneliness, 88
Low carbon buildings, viii, 55
Low-income, 32, 135
Low socioeconomic status, 85

M
Macro environment, 49
Man-Made Mineral Fibre (MMMF), 88, 99, 144
Marcus Vitruvius Pollio, 7
Mean radiant temperature, 51, 53, 89, 91
Medium environment, 49
Metabolic rate, 14, 51, 89, 123
Microbes-Volatile Organic (MVOC), 88, 104–106, 132, 133, 144
Microenvironment, 49
Mites, 107
Morphology, viii, 1, 10, 19
Moulds, 88, 104, 132
Multidisciplinary cooperation, viii, 34, 148
Multi-group interactions, viii, 83, 121, 140

N
Natural environment, 44
Naturally ventilated offices, 92, 129
Nearly zero-energy buildings, 24
Noise, 11, 12, 22, 25, 28, 31, 32, 46, 58, 60, 63, 67, 68, 84, 86, 87, 89, 92, 94, 123, 124, 127, 139

O
Occupants' perceptions, 50
Occupational stress, 88, 109
Odds ratio, 90
Odours, 61, 88, 96, 100, 110, 125, 127–129
Office dust, 107
Older people, 72
Opinion evidence, 28, 30
OR, 90, 138

Other indoor air pollutants, 88
Other risk factors, 87, 108, 134, 136
Overall comfort, 49
Ownership, 88, 110, 137
Oxidative stress, 109

P
Parameters related to building ventilation, 88
Personal factors, 90, 136–139
Phthalates, 88, 98, 99
Physical risk factors, 87
Physiological needs, 15, 48, 49
Plasticizers, 98, 106, 126
Polyvinyl chloride, 98, 126
Poor indoor air quality, 30, 32, 63, 97, 145
Population groups, 70
Preskar's cottage, 5, 6
Prevention and control, vii
Priority environments, viii, 43, 70
Probability, 59, 86, 90, 139
Problematic field, 140
Productivity, 27, 33, 34, 46, 50, 52, 56, 65, 69, 102, 103, 109, 145, 146
Psychosocial factors, 87, 88
Public and residential buildings, 43, 133
Public buildings, vii, 62, 70, 98
Public health and economic impact, 64
Public health strategies, 1
P-value, 90, 129
PVC, 98, 107, 126, 128, 130, 131

R
Radon, 31, 60, 66, 85, 97, 125
Recuperators, 27
Refurbishments, 24
Relative Risk (RR), 90, 91
Renovated buildings, vii, 29, 62
Renovation rates, viii
Risk assessment, 122
Risk factor, 85
Risk management, 122
Rodents, 88

S
Seasonal Affective Disorder (SAD), 69, 93, 95
Sick Building Syndrome (/-s), (SBS), vii, 60–62, 74, 89–92, 94–98, 100–110, 123, 124, 129–131, 134, 136–139, 146
Single group interactions, viii, 83, 121, 122, 140
Social status, 88, 134
Socrates's sun-tempered house, 5
Sound comfort, 49
Stakeholders, viii, 58

Stock of buildings, vii, 20
Study evidence, 27, 29, 30
Surface temperatures, 91, 127, 129, 143
Sustainable buildings, viii, 53
Symptomatology, 61

T
Terpenes, 100
Thermal comfort, 12, 19, 27, 30, 32, 33, 48–53,
        58, 88, 89, 123, 127, 129, 134, 135
Thermal environment, 49, 51, 52, 63, 65
Thermal performance, vii
Thermoregulation, 48
Total built environment, 2, 44, 45
Type of pollutants, 60, 87

U
Uncomfortable and unhealthy conditions, vii
Uncomfortable conditions, 49
Unhealthy and uncomfortable conditions, 1
Unhealthy built environments, viii
Unhealthy indoor environments, vii
Unilateral design, 147

Universal design, 95
User's opinions, 1
Utilitas, 7

V
Ventilation losses, 29
Venustas, 7
Vernacular buildings, 5
Vibrations, 88, 92, 123, 124, 127
Visual effects, 69, 92, 123
Volatile organic compounds (VOCs), 22, 60,
        66, 88, 96, 99, 100, 104–106, 125, 126,
        128, 130, 132, 144
Vulnerable population groups, vii, viii, ix, 30,
        43, 60

W
Wellbeing, viii, 1, 8, 19, 25, 26, 32, 43, 45, 47,
        53, 54, 56, 58, 59, 109, 121, 145
Winter mortality, 65
Worker performance, 146
Working position, 108
Work organization, 88

Printed in the United States
By Bookmasters